PRAISE FOR DR. ANNE MARIE MORSE AND *COMMUNICATION IN HEALTHCARE*

It's not by chance you picked up this book. It's a necessary tool for you to successfully navigate healthcare, irrespective if you are giving or receiving care. Let me share my experience with the gifted woman who authored it and references my family's journey in the beginning of this book.

Where do I begin? When God has destined a person to be connected by the circumstances of life, it is out of our hands. What can you do but go with the flow? Therefore, it was not left up to chance that my brother Shameen and I were at the right place at the right time to connect to Dr. Anne Marie Santilli (Dr. Morse's maiden name), Dr. K.I.R.D. (Keep it Real Doctor). Dr. Santilli will forever be a part of the Myers family.

I met Dr. Santilli in November 2012. My brother Shameen was transferred to Kings County hospital in Brooklyn, New York and Dr. Santilli was brought in to speak with us about my brother's diagnosis. Personally, I felt she looked too young to be so knowledgeable in the neurological field; mistake number one! Don't judge a book by its cover! From the onset, Dr. Santilli was clear, precise, knowledgeable, and compassionate, but I couldn't see it at that time. Mistake number two. I only saw that Shameen was sick. She is a doctor. Make my brother feel better. Mistake number three. I was selfish!

All the things that I considered negatives about Dr. Santilli, were actual blessings in disguise. Not only did she see, but she made the rest of the team see my brother as Shameen; me as Taffy—as Shameen's sister, not just his health care proxy; and our family as the Myers. She was and is the real deal. Every day, Shameen looked forward to seeing Dr. K.I.R.D. We were both disappointed when she was removed from his case . . . But she still came and saw us and never withdrew her compassion, sensitivity, and genuineness.

—Taffy Myers

My daughter, Makenzie, has been fortunate to have Dr. Anne Marie Morse on her healthcare team since the onset of a very complex illness. Dr. Morse's desire to truly listen to me, making me feel heard and understood, quickly set her apart from others. She influenced me to always be a strong advocate for my children. I am certain that this book will be a positive tool for physicians to improve their communication, as well as a great resource for patients and their caregivers who deserve to be heard.

—Nikki Shearer

Dr. Anne Marie Morse's *Communication in Healthcare* is a transformative guide to patient-directed care. By pioneering social listening, she takes an entrepreneurial approach to understanding her patients' needs and lived experiences—driving better health outcomes and setting a new standard for the medical community.

—Maria Picone
CEO, Trend Community

Anne Marie Morse, DO puts a new spin on patient-centered, results-oriented healthcare communication and empowerment. Anne Marie Morse's book is an easy read that reminds us why emotional intelligence is vitally important as a physician. *Communication in Healthcare* helps healthcare professionals and partners answer some of the most important questions that have emerged over the past year: How do I encourage patients and fellow physicians to empower themselves? How should physicians ensure optimal patient outcomes?

It's an absolute must read for any successful patient results in your medical career.

—Rachel Nesmith

Person living with narcolepsy with cataplexy

At just ten months old, my daughter Amity was in extreme agony. After several weeks of numerous doctor and ER visits, it was a singular interaction with Dr. Anne Marie Morse that led us to an immediate MRI of Amity's brain. Within just five hours, my husband and I were informed of life altering news. Amity would end up being diagnosed with a Grade III Anaplastic Ependymoma tumor. Dr. Morse began processing with us in every way possible—medically, emotionally, and mentally. I have no doubt that this book will be beneficial for healthcare partners, patients, and families alike to improve communication as it was such a vital tool—and sometimes a challenging task—for our family throughout Amity's treatment.

—Jackie Condor

Dr. Anne Marie Morse's book highlights the power of compassionate communication in modern healthcare. As medicine becomes more complex, strong patient-provider relationships are more important than ever. Through real-life examples, the author shows how good communication builds trust and improves care. A must read for healthcare professionals.

—Dr. Maria Sokolina
AADSM Diplomate
Host, Sleep Apnea: Breathing, Snoring Help

Healthcare is a journey that impacts all patients, family members, providers, and medical professionals. *Communication in Healthcare* is the road map where Dr. Ann Marie Morse guides you through the loops and turns of the communication barriers in healthcare. She encourages all members of the healthcare team to be active participants on this journey. She teaches how clear and intentional communication can empower patients and healthcare providers to be in the driver's seat on their journey and develop relationships built on trust, mutual respect, and teamwork, as well as provide meaningful change to each of their final destinations. Dr. Anne Marie Morse uses her medical knowledge, expertise, and her passion for caring for patients to help the reader find their inner strength and voice to navigate their personal health journey.

—Maggie Gary Lavender MSN, APRN, FNP-C

Communication in Healthcare: Charting the Course to Better Outcomes with Trust, Respect, and Teamwork is thought provoking and really embraces the idea of collaboration in order to achieve optimal outcomes. Dr. Morse is very passionate and has a genuine interest in supporting patients, improving lives, and ensuring benefit from the treatments being prescribed. She's able to present multiple strategies to consider, including some of the health behaviors, health literacy, cultural differences, and nuances that are expressed through a patient's body language and communication styles; all of which help inform the conversation and communication strategy, customized to the individual.

Dr. Morse brings not only years of experience to this book, but also provides clarity, direction, and thoughtful reasoning for people to consider and hopefully adapt some of the types of changes that they may want to consider in their own practice. She is sharing and translating her knowledge in a way that is easily disseminated and clearly driven by her passion to improve the lives of patients and population.

—Femida Gwadry-Sridhar, BSc Pharm, MSc (Epi), PhD
Chief Executive Officer and Founder, Pulse Infoframe

In *Communication in Healthcare*, Dr. Anne Marie Morse serves as your guide to the human aspects of the business of medicine. Healthcare providers and patients alike can rely on Dr. Morse's advice and look ahead to a year filled with ongoing learning, improved collaboration, and better results.

Dr. Morse is nothing short of a force of nature. She manages to be everywhere at once—caring for her patients with deep compassion, injecting passion and progress in the education and advocacy of Hypersomnia Disorders—all while authoring this indispensable guide to healthcare staff and leaders, and somehow making it all look effortless. From the moment I met her as my doctor, I knew I was in the best hands. She listens, she really cares, and she never stops fighting for better treatments and answers. Her dedication has changed my life, and I know I'm just one of so many who feel the same. The world of sleep medicine—and all of us lucky enough to be her patients—are better because of her.

—Tova DuPlessis

Founder, Essen Bakery

In today's increasingly complex, fast paced, and distracting healthcare system, Dr. Anne Marie Morse's brilliant new book reminds us of the critical importance of good communication if we truly wish to partner with the people we serve on their healthcare journeys. This is a must read and one which I guarantee you will reference over and over again for the wisdom and teaching pearls it contains.

— Dr. Mathieu Cuchanski

Neurologist and former neurology resident of Dr. Morse, who recognized her gift for healthcare communication and encouraged this book

Communication in Healthcare

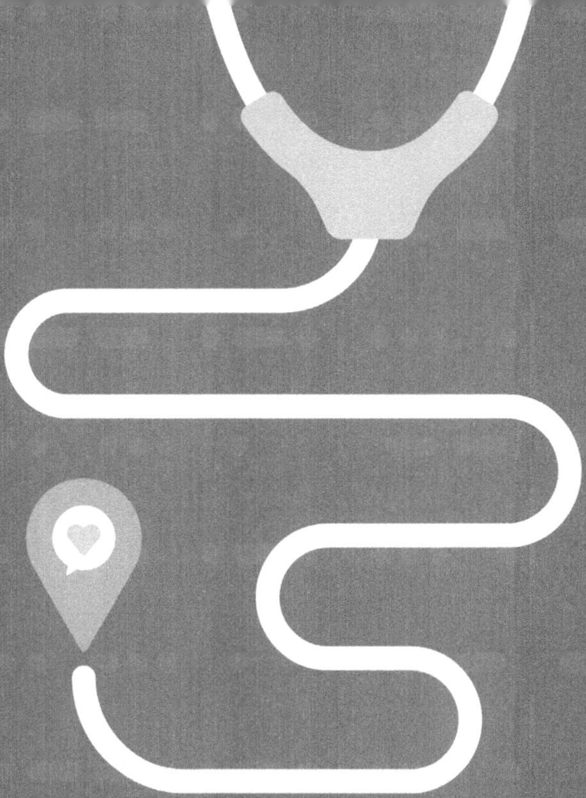

Anne Marie Morse, DO, FAASM

Communication in Healthcare

Charting the Course to Better Outcomes
with Trust, Respect, and Teamwork

Forbes | Books

Published by Forbes Books, Charleston, South Carolina.
An imprint of Advantage Media Group.

Printed in the United States of America.

10 9 8 7 6 5 4 3 2 1

ISBN: 979-8-88750-552-7 (Hardcover)
ISBN: 979-8-88750-553-4 (eBook)

Library of Congress Control Number: 2025902365

Cover design by Matthew Morse.
Layout design by Ruthie Wood.

04-15-2025 2:2

To my parents.

Thank you for teaching me the critical elements to becoming a leader, an advocate, and a changemaker.

And specifically, to my mother, who kept her diagnosis of multiple sclerosis invisible to others—a result of being left vulnerable to the belief that there were no therapeutic options for her, due to a failure of communication. My mission as a physician advocate and healthcare partner is dedicated to her.

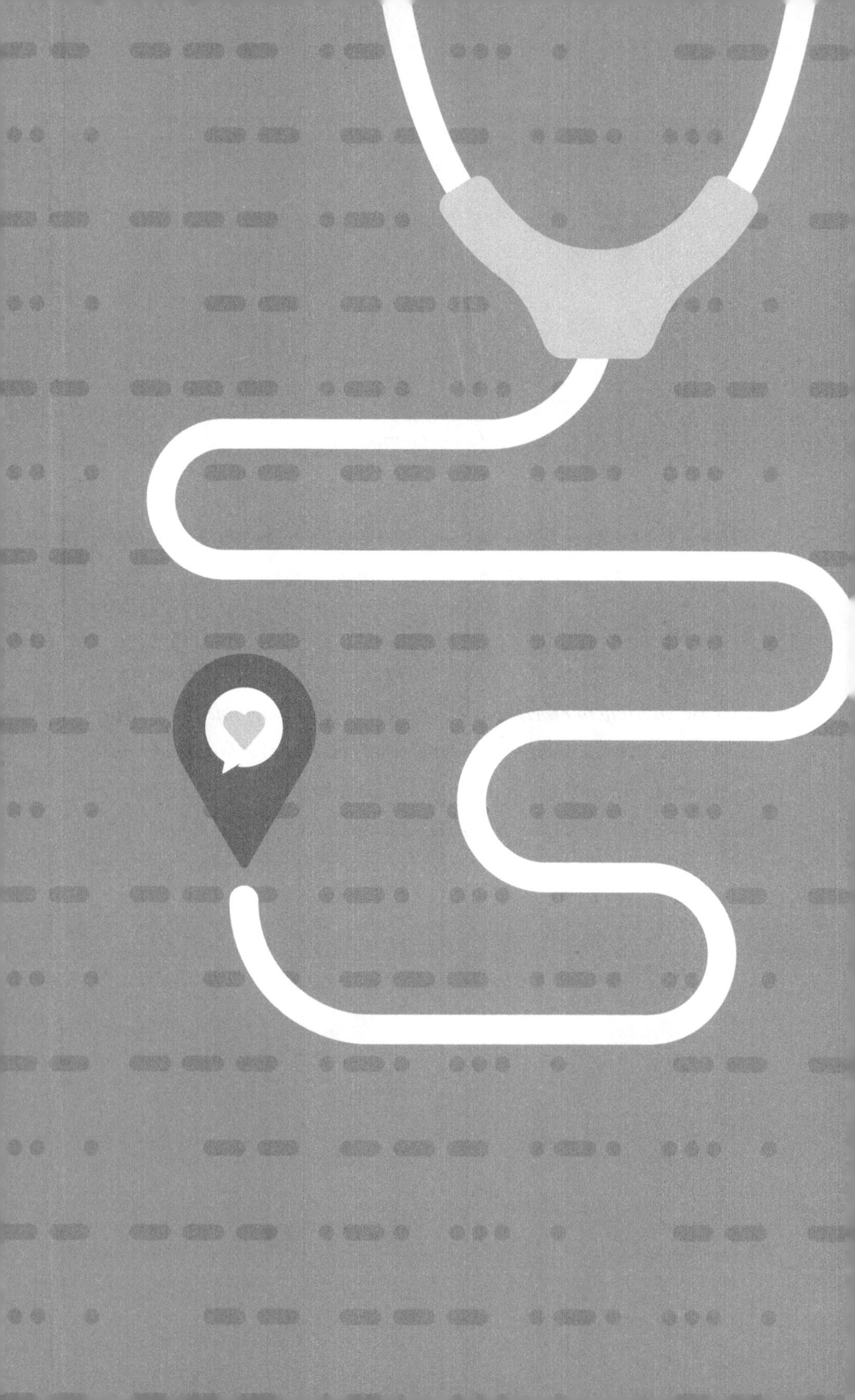

CONTENTS

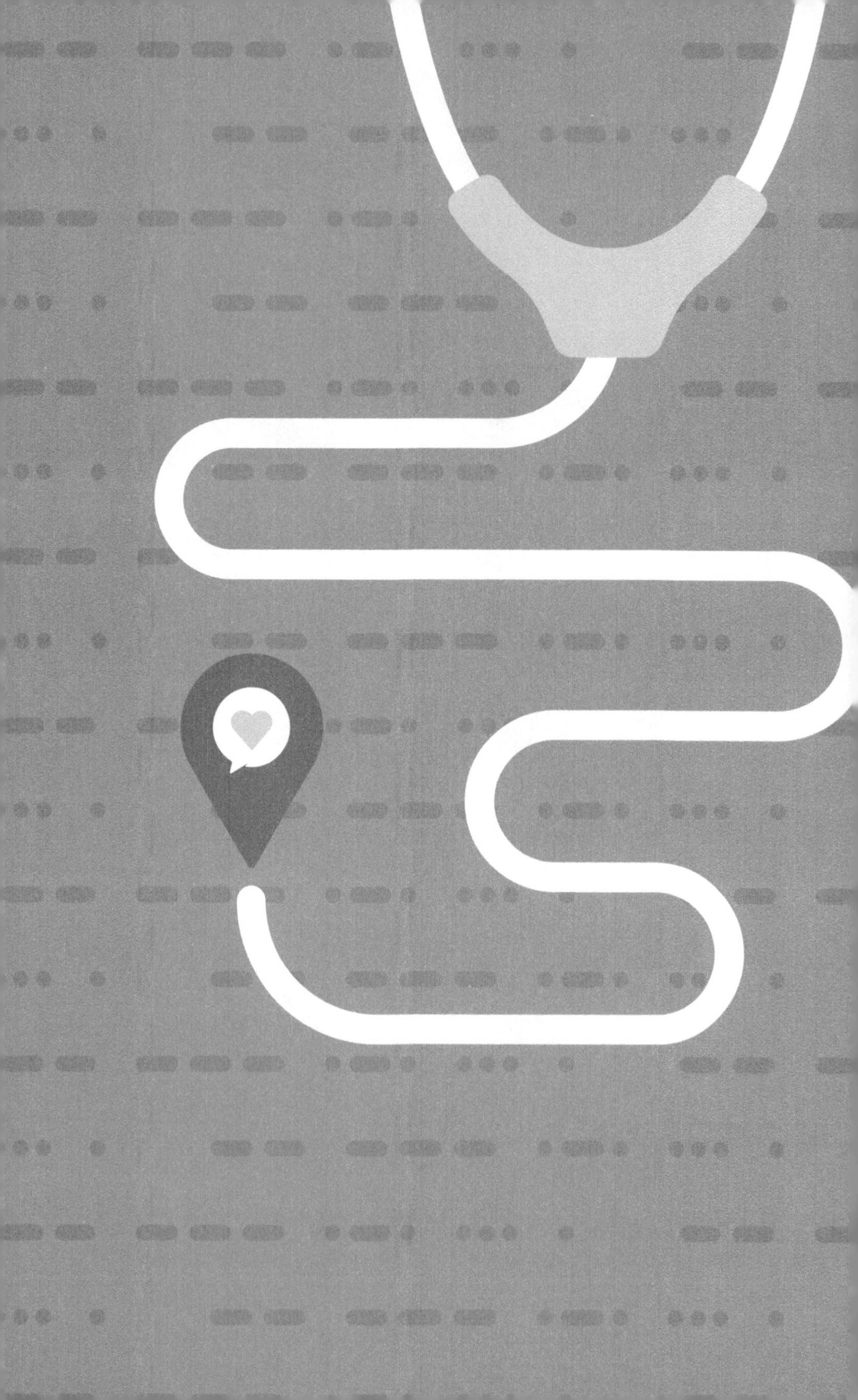

INTRODUCTION

Our Intention, Another's Perception

"During our first conversation, all I could think about was how much I hated you."

The family member of a patient I was treating admitted this to me a few weeks after we'd first met. Stunned, I went back over that initial interaction in my head. Where had my intention and her perception in that exchange diverged?

My first thought was how busy it had been at the hospital that night—one of those shifts when my pager seemed to go off with a critical emergency every minute. It was the first time I had been alone overnight as a first-year resident, or doctor in training, in neurology. On call, sleep-deprived, and stressed.

The patient, this family member's sibling, had been transferred to us following the identification of an aggressive brain tumor, a glioblastoma multiforme (GBM). It's one of the more common primary brain tumors in adults, and one of the most lethal. His family had brought him to the hospital for what they thought was a bad gastrointestinal bug—symptoms such as nausea, vomiting, and headaches.

The juxtaposition of an expectation of a viral illness versus the reality of a GBM, which at that time carried a prognosis of survival for six months to one year, was what I was left to convey.

As the on-call resident, I faced the need to be efficiently empathetic. I had to break this life-altering news to one family while trying to be present and lifesaving for another. In the middle of the night, I sat down with the patient's two sisters. Aware of the severity of the diagnosis, I made a conscious effort to be intellectually and emotionally present. However, I also wanted to be clear. I didn't want to sugarcoat the situation and give false hope. Simultaneously, during a busy on-call shift littered with stroke codes and other life-or-death scenarios, I needed to be concise. At the time, I was very junior in the medical pecking order, which also meant I had to choose my words wisely.

I sat with the patient's sisters, and we reviewed the MRI brain imaging acquired at the other hospital. I explained what we could and could not tell from those images: "This is what the pictures suggest, but we can't be sure until neurosurgery is able to intervene. We need to obtain tissue to confirm that this is truly what we think it is." I asked if they had any questions; they said no and that they would ask the nurses if anything came up.

Red flag. No questions? Unlikely. More likely, they were *so* overwhelmed by this information that they had a *million* questions. Another red flag: Had they suggested that they would speak with the nurses if something came up because they were hoping to avoid me or because they felt more comforted by the nurses? Maybe I should have offered to let them page me if further questions arose, or suggested that I could stop by again later.

I didn't note the red flags at the time. I left the room and went back to running around the hospital like a chicken with its head cut off, because it was *that* kind of night. If you're a physician or a nurse, you know the kind. And if you have ever had the unfortunate experience of being a patient or a family member of a patient in the hospital, you have probably witnessed some of this lunacy.

Several weeks later, I met with the patient and his sisters again. And that was when one of the sisters told me how she'd felt after that first exchange. While I had been going about my work, she had been sitting there, *hating* me. I remember her words distinctly: "I hated the words that were coming out of your mouth. I didn't want them to be true, so I hated you." Her sister, who hadn't had such a visceral reaction, told her, "You're just mad because she told us the facts. She didn't add sugar." This was true. I'd fed them a spoonful of vinegar, asked them to swallow it, and walked out of the room.

Could I have done anything differently? I couldn't have stayed with them all night to discuss the diagnosis. I was on call, with life-or-death situations playing out in other rooms of the hospital. But I *could* have taken the extra minute to assure them that they could ask me if they had further questions. I could have asked, "Are you OK?" or "Is there anything that I can help explain?" I could have acknowledged how hard it was to hear such information, especially when unexpected—this wasn't a virus that would go away in a few days but a GBM. I could have taken a second longer to recognize the expressions on their faces or the tenseness in their shoulders.

Unfortunately, this patient never left the hospital except for his own funeral. During this time, there was a complete reversal in my relationship with the family. The patient, "my boo," as I affectionately called him, found me to be a rock. I may have been low in the medical hierarchy, but I was the one he paged to come to his bedside when decisions were to be made about his care. His sister, who had initially hated me, found herself giving suggestions about my wedding planning. And during one of her brother's most difficult times, she handed me a letter to give to my now husband, thanking him for sharing me with the world to take care of those who needed me.

This incident took place over ten years ago. The sister who said she hated me? We are now friends. We even jokingly say we are "sisters from another mister." When my kids were born, she sent me handmade baby blankets. She texts me every Mother's Day, and periodically out of the blue: *I'm thinking of you. God bless you.* Clearly, she doesn't hate me anymore.

It was an eye-opening experience for me. I got a chance to come full circle with my relationship with "my boo" and his family. But that's not always the case. In most cases, a person who comes away from an unpleasant interaction in medicine is going to say, "I don't want to see that mean doctor [or nurse or whatever the title may be] again *ever*," and then they go find another professional. Second chances are not a given.

The saying that you only get one first impression is fact. Whether you are a doctor or a nurse, a patient or a family member, a caregiver or a member of a patient's broader community—the first interaction, especially when it comes to something as delicate as an individual's health, is critical. It has to be right the first time—and the time after that, and the time after that, and the time after that, since healthcare is an iterative process. If it's not right, we also need the skills to get it back on track.

That's what this book is all about: getting communication right. No more misaligned intentions/perceptions. Trust, respect, communication, best-in-class care, and teamwork—these are the core values that are foundational to excellence in healthcare. In medicine, providing care for people requires more than knowing medical textbooks inside and out, recognizing buzzwords, and getting good board scores. For patients and families, it requires more than knowing their own bodies and recognizing when something is "off." It requires keeping in mind that, at the core of each interaction, there is a person who is on a healthcare journey. Transparent, accurate, timely communication, not only confidently and clearly expressed but also listened to and acted on, is what will allow for the correct path forward. What are the steps we can take together, as a healthcare ecosystem, to make that possible?

The Web of Healthcare Communication

I am a board-certified and fellowship-trained adult neurologist with special qualifications in child neurology and sleep medicine. Since medical school, I have been invested in educating others. As a neurology resident (and although a Doctor of Osteopathic Medicine, DO), I was nominated and accepted into the allopathic (Doctor of Medicine, MD) medical honor society Alpha Omega Alpha based on having the following attributes: trustworthiness, character, caring, knowledge, scholarship, proficiency in the doctor–patient relationship, leadership, compassion, empathy, altruism, and servant leadership.

Education is a focal point of my career, and my commitment to teaching has grown with time, while the channels for its delivery have multiplied. I am an associate professor at the Geisinger Commonwealth College of Health Sciences, a distinguished educator in the Geisinger Academy of Educators, and the program director of the child neurology residency program at Geisinger, Janet Weis Children's Hospital. There is not an area of the healthcare ecosystem I have left untouched. I purposely invest my time in roles as an educator, speaker, adviser, consultant, investigator, and more—both nationally and internationally, and across multiple advocacy organizations, academies, and other healthcare sectors.

I also absolutely love educating and learning from the general public, which is why I started DAMM Good Sleep (DAMM as in my initials, Dr. Anne Marie Morse). This platform is focused on using sleep as a tool for prevention and wellness, and it capitalizes on communication to fill knowledge gaps, dispel medical myths, and learn about people's lived experiences—those not taught in textbooks—with different disorders. Name a social platform and you'll likely find DAMM Good Sleep on it, including TikTok. Yes, I'm one of those doctors you see on TikTok! No, you won't find me doing the latest dance craze; more likely, you'll find a quick, fact-filled message that raises awareness and educates.

Over the course of my career, I have encountered thousands of patients—as well as their friends, family members, and caregivers. I have also met countless other practitioners, including physicians, nurses, pharmacists, physical therapists, and others. Across all those interactions, a common theme has emerged when things have gone sideways: communication hurdles.

Make no mistake, I have had to learn from my own failures as well. Healthcare professionals spend years learning a new language—medicine—only to forget how to communicate with real people. People on their wellness journey expect to be safe while receiving care and to be able to trust the process and the people providing the care. However, that is with the presumption that everyone is on the same page—which is often not true.

The vicious cycle of misaligned communication is seen in burned-out providers, discouraged patients, poor outcomes, high costs of care, and overburdened, fragmented healthcare systems. Hospitals spend countless hours looking at point solutions—individual services designed to provide health, wellness, and/or condition-based services in the healthcare ecosystem—hoping to reduce costs, drive profit, and improve outcomes, many times without understanding how said solutions will communicate across the enterprise (and frequently without the input of key stakeholders such as staff, patients, or families). Meanwhile, failure to communicate properly is the driving force behind the dysfunction contributing to diagnostic error, lack of adherence, and poor outcomes.

As a physician, there have been plenty of times when I have been reminded to get out of my own way and rethink my communication approach. I recall a follow-up appointment with the parents of a child with epilepsy, a chronic seizure disorder. My words: "I have good news! The brain MRI is normal." The parents' response: "Great! So, he doesn't have seizures and doesn't need to take his medication anymore?" No; the medication was still very much needed! Some physicians may look at that conversation, slap their foreheads, and shake their heads in disbelief, blaming the patient for the erroneous response. However, I have learned to challenge that. I went through four years of medical school and six years of training to know what an MRI is, how it is used, and what it tells me. In this scenario, it was my failure that what I intended to say and what was interpreted were not the same.

In these instances, instead of choosing frustration, an emotion that conveys the idea that I cannot influence or change a situation or outcome, I choose to pursue the opportunity for improved communication—because this situation, and others like it, bring me back to the roots of why I became a physician: my mom.

I am the only doctor in my very large family, and it was my mom's healthcare journey that led me to medicine. Six months after she delivered my younger brother, her fourth child, she experienced her first significant clinical flare of multiple sclerosis (MS). She was in a wheelchair and had a dense hemisensory loss, which meant that she couldn't feel one side of her body and had corresponding weakness on that side. I don't remember any of this, as I was only five years old at the time. However, as I grew up, I witnessed her silent suffering, which often took shape as denial that she was living with a chronic disease. I witnessed her accounts of feeling vulnerable, with no solutions offered, and her feelings of being dismissed. I witnessed how she became discouraged and lost hope, with no healthcare partner she felt she could lean on. In light of her experiences, a career in medicine didn't become a choice for me but a must.

Imagine her experience: A stay-at-home mother, with four children—the youngest a newborn—experiences profound neurological symptoms. Following an initial medical evaluation, she is told it's a case of postpartum depression and that the symptoms will resolve when she isn't depressed anymore. Misdiagnosed and dismissed.

The reality? There were no depressed feelings, and her neurological symptoms persisted. Finally, a consultation with a neurologist, followed by a brain MRI and a spinal tap, revealed why: She had MS. She was given IV steroids for treatment, and her doctor told her, "If it gets better with steroids, great. If not, there's nothing more we can do." Or at least, that was her perception of what the doctor told her.

At the time, in 1989, no disease-modifying treatments for MS were clinically available. This was correct. However, there was still a need for a healthcare partner to provide support and surveillance. The doctor's lack of communication left my mother feeling abandoned. What she heard was that she could only look to herself for improvement and that she might as well go the rest of the journey alone. Thankfully, she did have a successful recovery after that flare. Still, over time, other subtle symptoms arose—foot drop, coordination problems, speech and swallowing difficulties. She "managed" these symptoms with a determination to overcome them, rather than by seeking and receiving appropriate medical evaluation and intervention.

Despite the continued flares, my mother went twenty years without seeing a neurologist. "There's nothing more we can do" haunted her. She did not want to feel dismissed, devalued, or devastated again. Instead, she lived in denial, frequently refusing to admit she had MS. Unfortunately, although advancements in MS treatment were made in the years following her diagnosis, she had no connection to physicians who could relay this to her. Because of a lack of hope and, perhaps, some element of fear, my mom became "lost to follow-up," not getting the subsequent surveillance and care she needed but making her healthcare journey alone.

Knowing my mother's experience, I made a promise to myself that when *I* became a physician, I would never let a patient or family travel their journey alone. I would always be empathetic and considerate in my interactions with patients and their families, so they felt supported and had the sense that we were in it together, even when it felt grim. And yet, decades later, there I was, having a patient's family member tell me: "During our first conversation, all I could think about was how much I hated you."

Somewhere along the way, I'd gotten caught in the tangled web of healthcare communication—which involves interactions not only between practitioners and patients but also among support staff, other providers, patients' families, caregivers, and broader communities. The more complex a disease, the more touchpoints it typically requires, the more specialists it demands, and the more complicated that web becomes. To untangle it, we first need to consider the perspectives of all those diverse players.

HEALTHCARE PARTNERS (THE NEW HCPS): THE MEDICAL EXPERTS

I use the term HCPs to refer to healthcare partners. Not healthcare providers, physicians, professionals, or practitioners. In my definition, a healthcare partner can be many things, not just a physician. HCPs may be doctors, nurses, physical therapists, psychiatrists, psychologists, pharmacists … The list goes on. Since my own perspective as an HCP is that of the physician, this is what I'll focus on for the moment.

My journey in medicine has been unique. I am a DO—an osteopathic physician—not an MD (or allopathic physician. As an osteopathic physician, the focus is always person first and disease second. This is reflected even in the way we are encouraged to talk about people. It's not "a hypertensive patient"; it's "Sarah, who has high blood pressure or hypertension."

My specific medical school training was likewise unique. In a traditional medical curriculum, you show up for the first two years and sit in a classroom, learn information, and take tests where you regurgitate that information. Generally, you learn physiology in your first year, which is how the body works, and pathophysiology in the second year, which is basically what happens when the body doesn't work as designed. In years three and four, you interact with actual humans in a supervised environment, such as a hospital setting.

My training was more person-focused from the beginning. I was one of five students selected for a problem-based learning model at Rowan University's School of Osteopathic Medicine. We would meet three days a week, for three hours a day, to discuss and learn from hypothetical patient cases. The remainder of the time was for independent learning. We would then return to the group and discuss the next steps on how to appropriately get to the right diagnosis and treatment for our hypothetical patient.

I remember my first day of medical school, when our group showed up and "met" Mrs. Meadows, our initial patient case study. Mrs. Meadows was a fifty-five-year-old woman who presented in the emergency room (ER) with increasing shortness of breath. We had to figure out what was wrong with her. At this point in our training, our knowledge of medicine was no different from that of most nonmedical professionals.

We started suggesting all the possible causes we could think of for Mrs. Meadows's shortness of breath. Whiteboards were set up, and we scribbled our thoughts on them to compile a differential diagnosis (a list of conditions that could explain Mrs. Meadows's symptoms) as well as any new information we collected about Mrs. Meadows to help guide that differential toward the most likely cause. Our facilitator was a guide on the side, listening and responding to make sure we didn't go off the rails. Mrs. Meadows was supposed to serve as our teacher, helping us to identify our knowledge gaps through her needs.

The process involved utilizing a series of books that allowed us to ask questions to the imaginary Mrs. Meadows, perform theoretical physical exams, and even run imaginary tests that could help us narrow down her differential diagnosis. As we collected information, asked questions, and considered differentials, we identified learning issues—things we didn't know. The list was vast. At the end of each session, each one of us would take responsibility for a learning issue, which we'd research before coming back and teaching it to the others in the next session. This method of learning resulted not only in the development of medical knowledge but also in emotional intelligence and an appreciation for a team-based approach to care.

It was in the context of that self-taught curriculum that Google became my best friend. In that first year, I became quite aware that I didn't know medical terminology. For instance, if our imaginary patient presented with yellowing of the skin and eyes, I'd google it and learn this was jaundice. No, Google was not my go-to for all my medical learning. But it was my go-to for learning how to find the information I needed *within* medicine. This experience helped me recognize the need to *translate* medical speak. It also taught me to avoid discouraging others who use Google to understand the language of medicine.

The teamwork required to get through those case studies also highlighted the importance of communication for me. Egos needed to be checked at the door. Emotions needed to be balanced. Focus needed to be maintained on *all* the words being used, to ensure we fully understood one another. Our education depended on it, as did the outcome for our hypothetical patient. Inevitably, there were disagreements about which references to use to support what we were saying, or what test should be ordered to support which diagnosis. However, we quickly learned that if someone felt disrespected or unheard, they shut down. The team then faltered, and we failed both in our learning and in serving our patient. It became clear that open, respectful communication was needed if we were to learn as individuals, thrive as a group, and do good for Mrs. Meadows and those like her.

Although the patients were imaginary, they were the focal point. It was through characters such as Mrs. Meadows that we learned the physiology and biochemistry of the lung, rather than by just reading about it in a textbook. A "person" was always at the center of our learning as we developed our medical expertise.

PATIENTS AND THEIR CAREGIVERS: EXPERTS IN THE PATIENT EXPERIENCE

Unfortunately, I think what ends up happening in many medical school and residency programs is that people are rewarded for knowing the jargon, to the point that they forget how to translate that jargon into simpler terms. Medical education is set up to positively praise individuals who select the right multiple-choice response to a question that is filled with buzzwords that signal the correct response. However, getting multiple-choice questions correct doesn't necessarily mean someone will be a good doctor. I have yet to meet a patient with the choices A, B, C, or D on their forehead to give me a hint what the right diagnosis or treatment may be. It has proven to be much more challenging to understand the lexicon used by a layperson to describe their lived experience, translate it medically to identify a diagnosis, and then provide a response—including a care plan—that can be mutually understood and agreed upon.

While HCPs may have trouble translating their expertise—medicine—for patients, we at least take some classes in school designed to address this communication gap. In contrast, a patient trying to express *their* expertise—their lived experience—doesn't take a class on how to do this and may therefore struggle when "translating" it for the HCP. There is no course, thesaurus, or similar resource to facilitate this. Even describing a symptom is a challenge, as the lived experience of that symptom can vary according to the individual. Pain is an excellent example. Everyone perceives pain differently—an issue that we've come up with all kinds of ways to try to address, such as scaled pain charts.

With this stated, there are steps patients can take to help improve the communication of their unique lived expertise to HCPs, such as keeping symptom diaries. We will talk about these tools in the chapters to come, while also considering the role that caregivers (family, friends, professional caregivers) may play. In the case of an ailment such as dementia, for instance, it may be not the patient themselves but a partner or caregiver who lives with them who can provide the most valuable insights into the patient's condition.

COMMUNITIES: THE BROADER CONTEXT

Comprehensive healthcare that is proactive, not just reactive, includes the community. Community can come in varied forms, from schools and churches to barbershops and beauty salons. If we really want to untangle the web of healthcare communication, the community must be considered.

The power of community should be leveraged. One of the programs I've developed, Geisinger's Wake Up and Learn®, is an example of what a difference community-based initiatives can make. Wake Up and Learn is a school-based sleep education and screening initiative for middle- and high school students that encourages a change culture around sleep health. Instead of perpetuating the "sleep when I'm dead" mentality or the idea of "getting away with less sleep," it promotes leveraging sleep as a tool to achieve outcomes that are important to teens, their families, and their schools. Sleep can help students in many ways, from enhanced mood stability to improved athletic performance and greater academic success.

Through its presence in the community, Wake Up and Learn provides screening and educational resources that help students become more autonomous and empowered, improving recognition of their own sleep problems and choosing the paths to address them. In the school district where we've been embedded the longest, we've seen students completely change their relationship with sleep, embracing it as a tool that helps them live the best version of themselves. After implementing the Wake Up and Learn program, the percentage of students experiencing problematic sleep steeply declined, from 64 to 38 percent.

This is just one example of the role community plays in filling the gap to achieve a continuous longitudinal model of healthcare optimization. Education, screening, and communication take many forms within the community. Imagine an individual unknowingly developing skin cancer and her hairdresser saying, "Hey, did you know you have a funny mole on the back of your neck? You should have that looked at by your primary care or dermatologist." Alternatively, consider a workplace that provides annual physical screenings in the office, or a church that destigmatizes seeking healthcare by sharing information about free public health initiatives. These bodies serve as a trusted bridge between the medical community and the local community. Making community-relevant resources and support available where people live, work, and socialize improves communication, facilitates the closure of care gaps, and helps achieve more optimal outcomes.

Putting the Patient in the Driver's Seat

Healthcare is a journey. Irrespective of whether a person is well, trying to navigate new symptoms, or living with a chronic disease—the patient should be in the driver's seat. This empowers them to set *their* preferred destination and determine the course of *their* journey. The HCP, with their medical expertise, can serve as the GPS—in this case, their Guiding Partner Specialist rather than their global positioning system. The patient should be able to input a destination into their GPS (say, a life free of XYZ symptoms) and the GPS should be able to tell them the possible routes to get there, how long it may take, any detours that may occur, and when they might need to completely reroute.

It is important to recognize that even the best GPS is only as good as the information it receives and integrates. In addition to the preferred destination, a GPS is constantly considering new information that may sometimes suggest an alternative route as a better choice. At times, this additional information may come from the driver. However, input from others in the patient's metaphorical car—from community members to partners—can be valuable, too. Perhaps, instead of the road sign saying, "Delays ahead because of debris in the road," this input could be a friend saying, "Hey, I noticed you haven't been eating much, and it looks like you may have lost some weight. Is everything OK?" Like the road sign may inspire a driver to pull over, this input may inspire a person to seek care. Or you could compare the community to a road crew cleaning up debris from the highway so people can drive safely without hazards. For example, this could be a school running vision and hearing tests to ensure its students can learn without impediment.

This book is intended to consider the care journey and *all* its participants, and it includes medical concerns from both sides of care: the delivering and receiving sides. You can read it cover to cover, or you can focus on those chapters that reflect where you are in your own care journey. Ultimately, the aim of this book is to put patients in the driver's seat. Once a person can confidently communicate with their HCP, they gain control of the steering wheel. They can then input information into the GPS, who can then ensure they reach their desired destination. The result? Improved patient satisfaction and outcomes, greater efficiency and professional satisfaction for HCPs, and reduced burden and cost within healthcare systems.

Each of the following chapters will open with a fictional narrative case study—an exchange between an HCP and a patient. The communication portrayed will provide an example of an instance where there has been a communication breakdown. We will then unpack that example and discuss the chapter's broader themes, including exercises to evaluate individual strengths and opportunities, system-based considerations, and solutions to the communication barrier we've just witnessed. The chapter will conclude with the same narrative case study but with an alternate ending, one in which the communication barriers have been addressed—and the patient outcome has changed as a result.

Given that each vignette will touch on a specific disease area, each chapter will also include a Community Support section, which will provide resources that HCPs, patients, and others can turn to if that disease is present in their lives. Recognizing that different people absorb information in different ways, I have attempted to make these resources diverse, ranging from social media accounts to printables, podcasts, YouTube videos, and beyond.

The book will also include checklists, exercises, and other tools designed to help both HCPs and patients to overcome communication barriers. Some resources are more patient-centric; others are more HCP-centric. Even if a resource doesn't speak to you directly, I encourage you to look at it and put yourself in the shoes of the intended target audience.

I didn't write this book just for patients or just for doctors. Besides, the line between the two is not firm. Every HCP has been a patient or a loved one of a patient at some point in their lives. And patients can become HCPs or community champions for care. We've all had a friend or family member touched by illness and stepped into the role of supporter or even caregiver. If we really want to fix the communication challenges in healthcare, we all need to come from a place of greater understanding for others. The first step? We could all use a higher EQ.

GROWTH OPPORTUNITY: WHAT'S YOUR DESIRED DESTINATION?

Borrowing from Dr. Seuss's *Oh, the Places You'll Go!*, examine where you are, where you want to be, and what you'll need to get there. This book is intentionally designed, so it is not exclusively for either HCPs or patients. It's meant to address communication across the healthcare ecosystem. Therefore, I encourage you to start by asking yourself, what is *your* place in that ecosystem?

Once you have identified your role, consider what additional contexts you may bring with you. Think about your education, background, training, biases, culture, etc., and how these might influence you in your role.

Finally, what is your intention with this book? Perhaps you are a physician who has noticed friction in patient communication. Perhaps you are a patient who is having difficulty conveying your symptoms to your HCP. Or perhaps you are the family member of a patient, watching them struggle and wanting to understand how you can help.

PROLOGUE

I did it. I got into medical school. I held the acceptance letter in my trembling hand. I was bursting with excitement and pride.

As I called my mom to share the news, an inkling of trepidation seeped in.

I already knew that I wanted to pursue neurology, so as soon as we were done celebrating, I told her, "I can't be the neurologist whose own mom has MS and doesn't see a neurologist. You have to go back to the doctor, Mom. You can't embarrass me."

My mom had spent most of her illness either denying that she had MS or joking about it—a coping mechanism. It was as though she had convinced herself that if she didn't acknowledge it, it didn't exist. Now I was asking her to face it. And although my statement about being embarrassed had been said half-jokingly, I hoped it would encourage her to act. I wanted her to find an HCP we could both trust and learn from. Most of all, I didn't want her to continue her journey alone. She dutifully went back to her neurologist.

When we got her MRI scans from that long-overdue follow-up visit, the images of her brain showed a great number of demyelinating lesions and black holes—MS-related lesions and a loss of brain tissue as a result. My mom, as usual, turned to humor: "My brain looks like a Swiss cheese!" But I felt incredibly sad.

To me, each of those lesions was an instance of my mom being lost to follow-up. The MRI showed years of injury because of a lack of treatment—treatment that my mom hadn't been aware of or hadn't understood well enough to see the point of … or, perhaps most heart-achingly, had been afraid to place hope in.

A patient who loses hope is a lost patient. Not just to follow-up but to care.

I do not want to see any more lost patients.

CHAPTER 1

Communication Starts with an *E*

The purpose of this chapter is to introduce the benefits and framework needed across the healthcare ecosystem for successful communication, as well as to examine the risks and repercussions when it fails. With that stated, it is only appropriate to ensure clear articulation of exactly what this book means by communication. Therefore, this chapter will define and review the different types and modes of communication, the various factors that influence the success of communication, and what can be done to improve it. In this chapter, we will lay out the foundation for ongoing skill building and for the changes needed to improve communication in order to achieve optimal outcomes: the emotional quotient (EQ)—sometimes referred to as emotional intelligence, or EI.

NARRATIVE CASE STUDY: A SLEEPY SOCCER PLAYER FIGHTS FOR FUNCTION

Jenny is seeing Dr. Jones for the first time. She is seeking help for her fatigue, which keeps her from playing soccer, a sport she enjoys. What Jenny doesn't know yet is that she has narcolepsy. Dr. Jones will need to pick up on Jenny's verbal and nonverbal cues if he is to diagnose her correctly.

I am exhausted. This is the third specialist I've seen this year to try to figure out what the hell is going on with me. Why am I so tired all the time? I dig my fingernails into my palms so hard that they leave little red crescent moons in my skin. I'm just trying to keep my eyes open.

"So, Jenny, what brings you in today?" Dr. Jones settles into the chair opposite me, a tablet in his hand. My tired eyes look at him with hope. Maybe *this* is the doctor who will finally figure out what's wrong with me.

"I'm just so tired all the time."

"Mmhm. Having trouble sleeping? For how long?"

"Over a year. I can't even play soccer, I'm so exhausted."

"Ah, I see, you're not doing activities you once enjoyed?" Dr. Jones's eyes light up and he starts scrolling through the tablet in his hand, as if searching for a solution. "I see here that ..."

He keeps droning on, but my eyelids are getting heavier and heavier. *I'll close them for just a second; he's not looking anyway ...*

"Jenny!" Dr. Jones's sharp voice startles me awake. He's obviously annoyed.

***

I can't believe my patient just fell asleep in front of me. I try to conceal my annoyance, reminding myself that she's ill—very likely depressed, based on what I've heard so far.

"I'm sorry!" She slouches down in her seat. "I didn't sleep well last night."

"I understand. Well, let's try to figure out what this is." I am careful to keep my tone friendly. If I'm going to diagnose Jenny, I need her to feel comfortable sharing with me. "Any other symptoms? Changes in diet? Exercise? Medication?"

"No. But I've started taking naps. I'm so tired during the day, all I want to do is sleep. I've gained weight. I've barely been going to work."

I nod, my suspicions growing stronger. I'm increasingly sure that Jenny has depression. As she continues speaking, I scroll through my tablet and review the digital intake form she completed before our meeting.

"Jenny, what I'd like to do is refer you to a psychiatrist. I think they may be able to help you."

"OK." The patient nods. I note the dark circles under her eyes, the unkempt hair, the ashen skin ... She certainly looks like she hasn't been sleeping much. I give her a sympathetic smile. An antidepressant should help.

I have spent much of my career devoted to the study and treatment of narcolepsy, a chronic neurological disorder that affects the brain's ability to control sleep–wake cycles. Unfortunately, this is also a disorder that is plagued by missed and misdiagnoses, resulting in severely delayed care. It can take as long as eight to twenty years from symptom onset to diagnosis.[1] The healthcare communication deficit is highlighted in the narcolepsy journey in unique ways, making this example a great entry point for discussion.

First, the lexicon being used often doesn't match the reality of what's happening. A doctor who is very familiar with the condition might hear Jenny's words in the opening scene and think "narcolepsy." However, I venture that many would hear the same thing as Dr. Jones—"I'm tired. I'm sleepy. I don't do the activities I used to."—and assume depression.

The doctor is hearing what the patient is saying, but he's also not *really* listening. For example, when the patient notes, "I can't even play soccer, I'm so exhausted," Dr. Jones thinks Jenny is describing anhedonia—a lack of interest in, enjoyment of, or pleasure from life's experiences. It's common in many mental health conditions, including depression. But it's not that Jenny doesn't enjoy soccer; it's that she's *too sleepy* to play.

We are also seeing a lack of EQ, demonstrated here by a lack of both self-awareness and social awareness. Dr. Jones is scrolling on his tablet. He is not observing the patient during the discussion and is thus failing to notice that she is struggling to keep her eyes open. At the end of the visit, Dr. Jones notices that Jenny looks sleepy, but at this point, this observation is only confirming the diagnosis he's already made: depression.

So, Jenny, who actually has narcolepsy, will be shuffled off to a psychiatrist, who may very well prescribe an antidepressant—which is likely to mask some of the symptoms of narcolepsy that Jenny may be experiencing, thereby further delaying her correct diagnosis. In the worst-case scenario, Jenny may give up hope and stop seeking help, becoming another patient lost to follow-up.

Healthcare Is Evolving, but Communication Remains a Problem

This kind of misdiagnosis is unfortunately common in narcolepsy. Jenny may find herself in the system, bouncing between specialists, for years. This adds to the burden on the healthcare system and, most significantly, leaves Jenny unable to lead the life she desires.

The biggest cost in such cases is the patient's quality of life. However, there are other costs, too. For instance, communication failures can lead to malpractice claims against physicians and health systems; one survey of malpractice claims identified communication failures in 49 percent of claims.[2] Communication issues can also be a factor in preventable adverse events, which can lead to poorer patient outcomes and patient suffering—and result in longer hospital stays and billions in additional healthcare spending every year.[3]

The risks of miscommunication—and the associated costs, both tangible and intangible—are becoming even greater in light of current changes to the healthcare landscape. Let's talk about that evolution.

Healthcare used to be based on a trusted relationship with the family physician, whom you visited in their office—or who perhaps even visited you at home—for as long as required. This is no longer the expectation but rather the exception. The primary care physician has been replaced by what feels like a revolving door of professionals.

Market forces are changing, as healthcare increasingly becomes a consumer business. I don't like to refer to patients as "consumers" because it takes away from the humanity of the healthcare interaction, but they are often seen and referred to in that way. We are seeing companies such as Amazon enter the healthcare space; in 2023, Amazon partnered with One Medical to provide primary care access to Amazon Prime members.[4] This is only one of the avenues the e-commerce giant has explored in entering the healthcare arena.

At the same time, we are facing an increasing complexity of care. Today, we can analyze patients at the molecular level. Fifty years ago, it would have been unthinkable for a woman to undergo a risk-reducing mastectomy following the identification of a BRCA1 gene mutation (which indicates a predisposed risk for breast cancer). Now this procedure has made headlines, in part thanks to celebrities such as Angelina Jolie, who wrote an op-ed on her choice for *The New York Times* in 2013.[5]

There are also technological advancements that are impacting healthcare. Take something as simple as a tablet, like the one Dr. Jones has in our narrative case study. A tablet can make so many tasks easier for an HCP, providing an on-the-go, searchable, organized database of information, from a patient's medical history to what tests have been ordered for them. But a tablet can also be a distraction in a patient–provider interaction and, one might argue, detract from the humanity of such encounters: Dr. Jones isn't even making eye contact with his patient as he speaks to her. In a similar vein, I have seen hospitals replace in-person check-ins with automated kiosks, like you'd use to order your hamburger at McDonald's. Again, the commodification—or consumerification—of healthcare comes to mind.

Of course, tech in healthcare isn't all bad. It can also be beneficial. Apps can help patients record symptoms, manage medications, and track lifestyle factors such as exercise sessions, sleep and wake times, and mindfulness practices. Tracking these things can be a valuable first step in behavior modification, which is often necessary for general wellness—especially for a complex condition such as narcolepsy.

There are also more complex technologies entering healthcare, such as machine learning (ML) and artificial intelligence, that can have great benefits. In the case of narcolepsy, for instance, ML may be useful in enhancing diagnostics. The typical approach to diagnosing narcolepsy is to do an overnight sleep test, called a polysomnography, followed by a next-day multiple sleep latency test (MSLT). The MSLT is really the test that will diagnose narcolepsy. However, ML models have been applied to overnight polysomnography and have been shown to have the same diagnostic sensitivity and specificity as the MSLT, if not superior.[6] Faster, more accurate, more cost effective—this is a great example of technology benefiting patients, HCPs, and systems alike.

What Does Communication in Healthcare Look Like Today?

What do we mean by communication, anyway? I have found this definition of communication, seen in various academic contexts, useful: "Communication is the process of generating meaning by sending and receiving symbolic cues that are influenced by multiple contexts."[7] Scholarly articles on communication tend to identify five different forms:[8]

- **Intrapersonal communication** occurs within oneself, from the thoughts in your head to perceptions of internal sensations, such as a rising heart rate.
- **Interpersonal communication** occurs between people (usually two) whose lives mutually influence one another, such as an HCP and a patient.

- **Group communication** occurs between three or more people communicating to achieve a shared goal. My med school program of students collaborating to diagnose imaginary patient case studies is an example.
- **Public communication** usually consists of one person conveying information to an audience. The TikTok videos I disseminate through DAMM Good Sleep are an example.
- **Mass communication** occurs when messages are sent to large audiences. In the healthcare space, this could look like public health information—say, websites about health topics.

As healthcare has evolved, so has the communication around it. As we go on to unpack communication barriers and how to overcome them, I want to touch on the key points that I've seen influence communication in the healthcare space.

TYPES OF COMMUNICATION

Communication can be broken down into verbal and nonverbal. More specifically, this can look like:

- **Spoken words:** This refers not only to the content of the words but also the tone they are delivered in and the vocabulary used. Consider the impact of using medical jargon versus layperson's terms.
- **Body language:** Spoken words are supported by body language, including facial expressions, gestures, and posture. Something as simple as crossed arms can say a lot.
- **Written words:** For the written word, content and vocabulary are likewise relevant. In this case, "style" might replace the

idea of "tone." A flowery, long speech is perceived differently than one that's plainspoken and to the point.

- **Visual images:** Communication via imagery is also possible and can convey a mood (similar to a tone or a style). Think of how a pediatrician's waiting room looks versus the waiting room of a general practitioner for adults.

How the type of communication is presented matters. Want proof? A study of healthcare-related responses on a public online form, including questions about diagnoses, compared how people perceived responses from ChatGPT versus responses from physicians. People found the ChatGPT responses more empathetic and of better quality because ChatGPT provided more flowery, lengthier responses. However, ChatGPT also provided information that was factually incorrect. The ChatGPT responses weren't "better"; they were just presented in prettier packaging.[9] Presentation matters.

MODES OF COMMUNICATION

These days, there are more modes of communication available to us than ever before. As technology advances, odds are that we'll have even more options in the future. For now, we've got:

- **In-person:** Face-to-face interactions are still a cornerstone of healthcare. Diagnosis, treatment, and care are often only possible with in-person intervention.
- **Telephone:** Phone calls allow for the same direct and immediate back-and-forth exchange as an in-person interaction. However, they lack the body language component.
- **Text and email:** Text and email remove the immediacy of in-person or telephone exchanges. The communication

becomes asynchronous, with each party responding in their own time frame.

- **Live chat:** Live chat, for instance via websites or apps, brings the immediacy back to written exchanges. There is the expectation of an immediate response.
- **Video:** Video-based consultations became more common during the COVID-19 pandemic and remain in use. This medium allows for immediate back-and-forth exchanges, supported with visuals.

On one hand, the proliferation of communication options creates complexity. On the other hand, it creates opportunities. For example, research suggests that telemedicine can be useful in improving mental healthcare in rural communities, where in-person access may not be possible.[10] It's even been shown to be as effective as in-person care in these communities.[11]

COMMUNICATION CONSIDERATIONS

Finally, there are many different factors that influence communication, both how it is given and how it is received—or intended and perceived. This list is just a starting point:

- **Language:** HCPs and patients don't always speak the same language, requiring interpretation.
- **Lexicon:** Even if they speak the same language, HCPs and patients don't necessarily share a lexicon. The vocabulary they use to describe a symptom may vary. Consider also how this changes in the case of a pediatric patient, whose lexicon is more limited.

- **Culture:** Culture is comprised of so many things, from food to dance—and even how we approach healthcare. Think of those home remedies you inherited from your mother or grandmother, for instance.
- **Religion:** Religion can impact all kinds of healthcare decisions, from whether a person is willing to have an abortion to whether they are willing to accept a blood transfusion.
- **Socioeconomics:** Finances impact when patients seek care. An annual checkup isn't a priority when money is tight. Unfortunately, this means some patients only get help when an ailment is well progressed, making it harder (sometimes impossible) to treat.
- **Technology access:** Not everybody has the same access to technology, for various reasons (socioeconomic, cultural, religious). As tech becomes more interwoven in how we provide care, access issues need addressing.
- **Health literacy:** Some patients may have a greater degree of health literacy than others. A nurse, for example, has more medical knowledge than a non-nurse. There is also the question of basic literacy, which is not a given.
- **Explicit/implicit bias:** This topic deserves its own book, and I cannot do it justice in these brief lines. I would like to flag it nonetheless and note that many excellent books have been written on the issue. One starting point: *Dismissed: Tackling the Biases That Undermine Our Health Care*, by Angela Marshall with Kathy Palokoff.[12]

All of these things add up to a greater context—a context that an individual brings with them to any communication interaction. I remember treating Haitian patients who would place a circular thread on a newborn baby's forehead to ward off the evil eye. The first time I witnessed this as a young resident, I thought the thread was a stray from the baby blanket that had landed on the baby's forehead accidentally, and I brushed it away—much to the mom's distress! A prime example of why cultural understanding is so pivotal.

If we take all the above and try to break it down into a simple visual, the complexity of the problem becomes apparent.

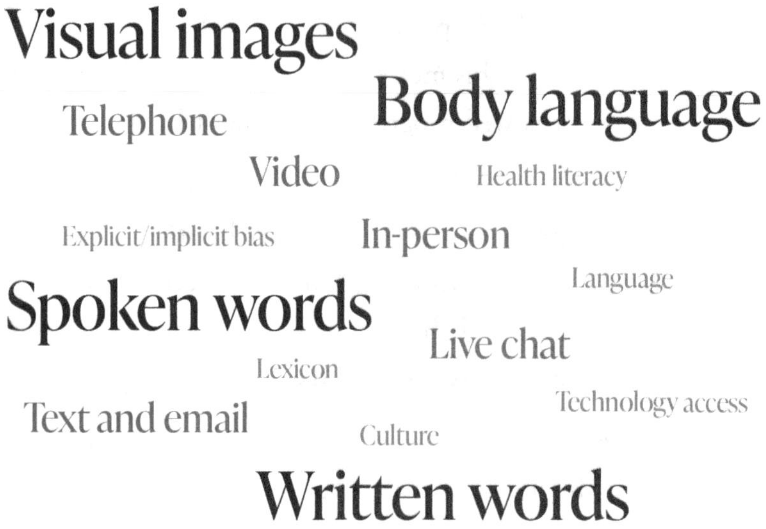

Figure 1.1: The many factors that influence communication in healthcare.

Looking at Figure 1.1, it becomes increasingly clear why communication in healthcare is difficult! There are so many factors at play, from different modes of communication to the personal contexts each person brings to any interaction.

Communication Callout

Throughout the book, you'll see callout boxes—like this one—entitled Communication Callout, each flagging some sort of communication consideration. A lexical consideration might focus on a pediatric patient with a limited vocabulary, for example, while a technological consideration might focus on a patient who lacks access to telemedicine tools.

Can this book solve it all? No. But it may help to recognize how these pieces impact intention–perception alignment. Recognizing the misalignment of intention versus perception can solve many communication problems—not all of them, but it's a start.

Emotional Quotient: The Baseline for Good Communication

In recent years, there has been a lot of buzz around value-based outcomes (VBO) in healthcare. In the VBO delivery model, providers are paid based on patient health outcomes. Proponents suggest that this encourages a more holistic approach to patient care, and there are certainly valid arguments for this model. However, the "value" in VBO models is based on measuring health outcomes against the cost of delivering those outcomes.[13] The focus is fiscal.

Take the example of a hospital attempting to improve care by using digital technologies. In a VBO model, the effectiveness of those technologies is often measured only against cost and quality (patient outcome) indicators. However, less is known about the clinician and patient experience. This is counter to previously accepted frameworks, such as the quadruple aim, which considers four goals: clinician experience, improved patient experience, improved population health, and reduced healthcare costs.[14]

I thus propose an alternative to VBO models: patient-valued outcomes. Does the outcome provide value to the patient, as defined by the patient? This brings us back to the idea of the patient as driver and the HCP as GPS—Guiding Partner Specialist. For that GPS to work, communication is key. And technology alone cannot fix the communication failures we are already seeing in healthcare—not if we continue to neglect the human element of care and, more specifically, the EQ.

EQ is the ability to understand and manage your own emotions, as well as to recognize and respond to the emotions of others.[15] The foundational elements of EQ are as follows:[16]

- **Self-awareness:** Exercising awareness of one's own feelings, motives, and desires.
- **Self-management:** Exercising control in how one responds to influences, both internal and external.
- **Social awareness:** Recognizing intentional and unintentional communication by another, empathizing with them, and considering alternative perspectives, especially those of people of different backgrounds and cultures.
- **Social management:** Acting in a socially aware way and considering alternative perspectives, especially those of people of different backgrounds and cultures.

There is a need to pay attention to yourself and to the other person. If you're practicing EQ, you'll be able to better regulate the gap between intention and perception.

The impact of EQ has been researched. For instance, one review found that EQ plays a significant role in the academic success of clinical year medical and dental students. Although this review addresses different rungs of the healthcare profession separately, it preludes the idea that better EQ skills in a healthcare team will have a holistic impact on healthcare improvement.[17] A different study examining patients with chronic lower back pain suggested that physician empathy improves patient outcomes.[18] And other research has indicated that physician EQ enhances patient satisfaction.[19]

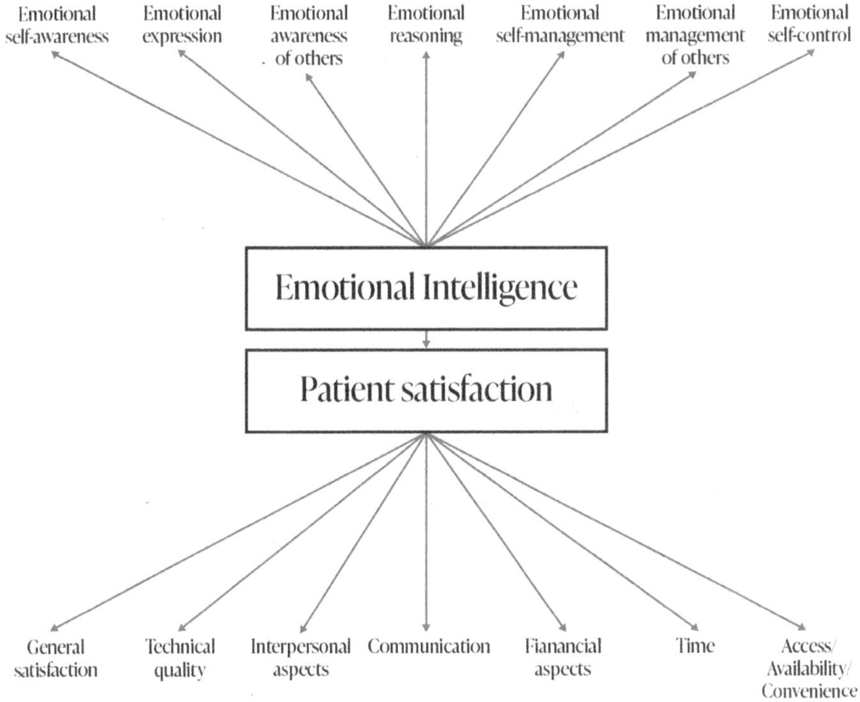

Figure 1.2: This graph is adapted from a study on physicians' EQ and patient satisfaction and shows how the two relate.

In my experience, good communication, rooted in EQ, progresses medicine beyond the reactive. When medicine is reactionary, people start making correlations that may not be causations, and they can end up stepping backward instead of moving forward. This contributes to distrust and discomfort in the delivery and receiving of care.

A NARRATIVE CASE STUDY, REIMAGINED

Our narrative case study of Jenny and Dr. Jones is one example of the difference EQ can make. What if the exchange we saw in the introduction had more self-awareness on both sides?

I am exhausted. This is the third specialist I've seen this year to try to figure out what is going on with me. Why am I so tired all the time? I dig my fingernails into my palms so hard that they leave red crescent moons in my skin. I'm just trying to keep my eyes open.

"So, Jenny, what brings you in today?" Dr. Jones settles into the chair opposite me, a tablet in his hand. I look at him with hope. Maybe *this* is the doctor who will finally figure out what's wrong with me.

"I'm just so tired all the time."

"Mmhm. Having trouble sleeping? For how long?"

"Over a year. I can't even play soccer, I'm so exhausted."

"I see. Is it that you don't enjoy the sport anymore? Or you're physically too tired to participate?" Dr. Jones leans forward, curious, his eyes on my face.

I can feel my eyelids getting heavier, and I want to stay focused, so I sit up straight and take a deep breath of oxygen into my lungs and tell him: "I love playing soccer! I want to play again regularly. That's my goal. But the fatigue makes it impossible."

***

I put my tablet to the side and observe the woman in front of me. She has dark circles under her eyes, her hair is unkempt, and her skin is ashen. She looks like she hasn't slept in days. Is it depression? Or something else?

"Let me just review what tests you've had in the past. If you'll give me one moment while I check your record." I pick up my tablet and read through, before putting it back down and returning my attention to Jenny.

"I see you had your thyroid checked, and that was normal."

"Yes, my other doctor thought that could be the reason for the fatigue. I also saw an infectious disease specialist because they thought I might have mono."

"It's good to rule those things out. I've noticed that you're having trouble keeping your eyes open." I note that she keeps digging her fingernails into her own hands, as if she's trying to pinch herself awake.

"Yeah, I have trouble staying awake at work, in class, even over dinner." She looks at me with despair.

This doesn't seem like regular depression, I think to myself. I ask Jenny questions about her sleep habits and patterns—until I realize something.

"Jenny, I can't say for sure, as we'd have to run some tests, but I think you may have narcolepsy. Have you heard of that condition?"

Her face brightens. "Yes! I actually googled my symptoms once and that came up." Her relief is evident.

"OK, like I said, I can't know for sure just yet. But let's get you set up with some tests to see."

Notice the greater attention to the other person? The self-awareness on both sides? Jenny knows she is about to drift off; she takes a deep breath and fills her lungs with oxygen. Dr. Jones knows he has to give his attention to his patient; he focuses on her, not his tablet.

Now Jenny will get an accurate diagnosis. Consider how drastically this could change her healthcare journey, especially keeping in mind that narcolepsy can take eight to twenty years to diagnose following the first presentation of symptoms. We've gone from A to B without all the in-between stops to see other HCPs and specialists.

This is the difference that can come from putting the patient in the driver's seat. I have seen the impact firsthand. I trained under Dr. Michael Thorpy, an internationally recognized expert in narcolepsy and idiopathic hypersomnia, at a time when his team was running a pediatric extension trial of a specific medication for the treatment of narcolepsy. Through that trial, I saw firsthand how the correct diagnosis—coupled with a treatment option—could change patients' lives. The parents of the children in the study would cry tears of joy when they realized that, after years of feeling helpless watching their kids struggle, they finally had answers.

COMMUNITY SUPPORT

The community can play a pivotal role in any healthcare journey. Social support becomes even more important in the case of rare diseases, such as narcolepsy, that may be prone to issues such as misdiagnosis and lack of awareness. Advocacy organizations and patient groups can be wonderful resources.

In the narcolepsy space, one resource I'd like to flag is **Wake Up Narcolepsy (WUN)**, a national nonprofit that has been empowering individuals and communities since 2008. They exist to drive awareness and education with goals that include reducing time between symptom onset and diagnosis and ensuring improved, accessible treatments. WUN offers several unique virtual support groups and in-person events and has contributed millions toward clinical research in the narcolepsy space.

Another resource is my company **DAMM Good Sleep**, which is designed to transform the role of sleep health in medicine. I frequently jest that I put the DAMM in DAMM Good Sleep (**D**r. **A**nne **M**arie **M**orse). DAMM Good Sleep is also my social media handle across platforms (TikTok, Instagram, X, Threads, Pinterest). I took to social media to learn from patients' lived experiences and to help augment individual access to education. My aim is to support empowered individuals on their journeys while also combating the misinformation and myths pervasive across social channels. I now have a growing number of Sleep Friends helping me contribute to the change, demonstrating the value of community.

Although we do not have all the answers yet, resources such as those above can help. They are also a reminder of the fact that healthcare done well is not just a result of effort by the patient or the HCP. In its best forms, healthcare is a community effort, one in which different parties take responsibility for their roles. Of course, the key players are the patient and the HCP, and as in any good relationship, accountability is needed on both sides.

Growth Opportunity: How's Your EQ?

Is EQ *the* answer to all of the communication challenges we face in healthcare? No. But I do believe it is the basis for good healthcare communication, especially in an ever-evolving landscape. Before we continue to some of the solutions for communication breakdown, figure out your baseline. How is your EQ? Scan the QR code for a self-assessment that can tell you.

Chapter 1 Endnotes

1 Erin C. Golden, MD, and Melissa C. Lipford, MD, "Narcolepsy: Diagnosis and Management," *Cleveland Clinic Journal of Medicine* 85, no. 12 (2018): 959–969, https://doi.org/10.3949/ccjm.85a.17086.

2 Kate E. Humphrey, Melissa Sundberg, Carly E. Milliren, Dionne A. Graham, and Christopher P. Landrigan, "Frequency and Nature of Communication and Handoff Failures in Medical Malpractice Claims," *Journal of Patient Safety* 18, no. 2 (2022): 130–137, https://doi.org/10.1097/PTS.0000000000000937.

3 Richard R. Hurtig, Rebecca M. Alper, and Benjamin Berkowitz, "The Cost of Not Addressing the Communication Barriers Faced by Hospitalized Patients," *Perspectives of the ASHA Special Interest Groups* 12, no. 3 (2018): 99–112, https://doi.org/10.1044/persp3.SIG12.99.

4 "Amazon Takes Another Shot at Health Care, This One a Virtual Care Service That Costs $9 Per Month," The Associated Press, November 9, 2023, https://apnews.com/article/amazon-medical-membership-b961a006c24f82a839f971708b609800.

5 Angelina Jolie, "My Medical Choice," *The New York Times*, May 14, 2013, https://www.nytimes.com/2013/05/14/opinion/my-medical-choice.html.

6 Jens B. Stephansen, Alexander N. Olesen, Mads Olsen, Aditya Ambati, Eileen B. Leary, Hyatt E. Moore et al., "Neural Network Analysis of Sleep Stages Enables Efficient Diagnosis of Narcolepsy," *Nature Communications* 9, no. 5229 (2018), https://doi.org/10.1038/s41467-018-07229-3.

7 Victoria Leonard, "Types of Communication" in *COMS 246: Interpersonal* Communication, course materials (College of the Canyons), accessed December 4, 2024, https://socialsci.libretexts.org/Courses/College_of_the_Canyons/COMS_246%3A_Interpersonal_Communication_(Leonard)/1%3A_Introduction_to_Communication/1.1%3A_Types_of_Communication.

8 Leonard, "Types of Communication."

9 John W. Ayers, Adam Poliak, Mark Dredze, Eric C. Leas, Zechariah Zhu, Jessica B. Kelley et al., "Comparing Physician and Artificial Intelligence Chatbot Responses to Patient Questions Posted to a Public Social Media Forum," *JAMA Internal Medicine* 183, no. 6 (April 2023): 589-–596, https://doi.org/10.1001/jamainternmed.2023.1838.

10 Jun Watanabe, Hiroyuki Teraura, Akihisa Nakamura, and Kazuhiko Kotani, "Telemental Health in Rural Areas: A Systematic Review," *Journal of Rural Medicine* 18, no. 2 (April 2023): 50–54, https://doi.org/10.2185/jrm.2022-059.

11 Carly McCord, Fred Ullrich, Kimberly A. S. Merchant, Divya Bhagianadh, Knute D. Carter, EveLynn Nelson et al., "Comparison of In-Person vs. Telebehavioral Health Outcomes from Rural Populations Across America," *BMC Psychiatry* 22, no. 778 (2022), https://doi.org/10.1186/s12888-022-04421-0.

12 Marshall, Angela. *Dismissed: Tackling the Biases that Undermine Our Health Care.* S.l.: CITADEL PR, 2024.

13 "What Is Value-Based Healthcare?" *NEJM Catalyst,* January 1, 2017, https://catalyst.nejm.org/doi/full/10.1056/CAT.17.0558.

14 Oliver J. Canfell, Leanna Woods, Yasaman Meshkat, Jenna Krivit, Brinda Gunashanhar, Christine Slade et al., "The Impact of Digital Hospitals on Patient and Clinician Experience: Systematic Review and Qualitative Evidence Synthesis," *Journal of Medical Internet Research* 26 (March 2024): e47715, https://doi.org/10.2196/47715.

15 J. D. Mayer, P. Salovey, D. R. Caruso, and G. Sitarenios, "Emotional Intelligence as a Standard Intelligence," *Emotion* 1, no. 3 (2001): 232–242, https://doi.org/10.1037/1528-3542.1.3.232.

16 Richard E. Boyatzis, Daniel Goleman, and Kenneth Rhee, "Clustering Competence in Emotional Intelligence: Insights from the Emotional Competence Inventory," in *The Handbook of Emotional Intelligence: Theory, Development, Assessment, and Application at Home, School, and in the Workplace,* eds. R. Bar-On and J. D. A. Parker (Jossey-Bass/Wiley, 2000).

17 Nikhilesh Singh, Sweta Kulkarni, and Richa Gupta, "Is Emotional Intelligence Related to Objective Parameters of Academic Performance in Medical, Dental, and Nursing Students: A Systematic Review," *Education for Health (Abdingdon)* 33, no. 1 (2020): 8–12, https://doi.org/10.4103/efh.EfH_208_17.

18 John C. Licciardone, Yen Tran, Khang Ngo, David Toledo, Navya Peddireddy, and Subhash Aryal, "Physician Empathy and Chronic Pain Outcomes," *JAMA Network Open* 7, no. 4 (2024): e246026, https://doi.org/10.1001/jamanetworkopen.2024.6026.

19 Shama Kadadi and Shankargouda R. Bharamanaikar, "Role of Emotional Intelligence in Healthcare Industry," *Drishtikon: A Management Journal* 11, no. 1 (October 2020): 37, https://www.researchgate.

net/publication/344955693_Role_of_Emotional_Intelligence_in_Healthcare_Industry.

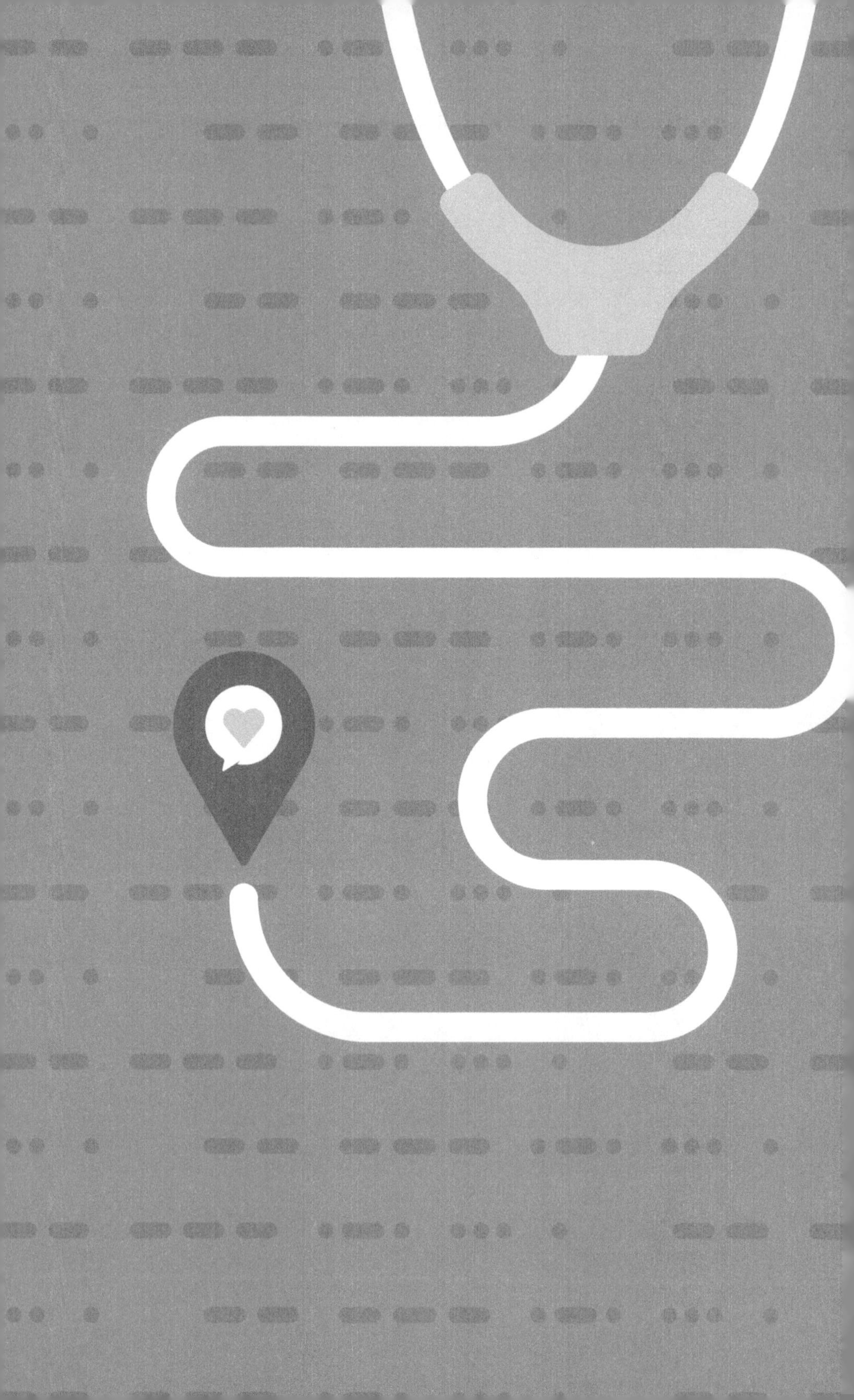

CHAPTER 2

A Perfect Partnership Needs Accountability

While we can create the expectation for accountability, we cannot make others accountable. The only person's actions you can control are your own. The purpose of this chapter is to introduce a system of self-reflection, a way to explore your own self-awareness and self-management. Do you recognize your own feelings, motives, and desires (self-awareness), and can you control how you respond to them (self-management)? The goal is to implement ongoing quality improvement to achieve the greatest degree of growth and consistency in these skills, reducing friction and improving clarity.

NARRATIVE CASE STUDY: A CONCERNED PERSON WITH CANCER SEEKS CLARITY

Carlos has recently been diagnosed with colon cancer, caught during a routine screening after his fifty-fifth birthday. Now he needs to find an oncologist to help him understand his diagnosis and prognosis and to provide him with a treatment and care plan. He has his first appointment with the oncologist his primary care physician referred him to today.

I'm terrified. Stage three colon cancer. Does this mean I'm going to die? My mouth is dry as I approach the reception desk at the doctor's office.

"Morning." The girl behind the front desk doesn't look at me.

"Good morning. I have an appointment with Dr. Williams." I slide my insurance card across the desk. I have a copy of my referral in my hand. I have everything I need, I think.

"Fourth floor is oncology. Check in there." Her tone is bored.

"Oh." I slide my insurance card back toward me and look around for an elevator. After walking down one wrong hallway and then another, I find it and make my way upstairs.

The receptionist on the oncology floor is friendlier and checks me in quickly. But there's an issue with my insurance: "It looks like you haven't met your deductible for the year." *Crap.* I reach for my credit card.

Now all I have to do is wait. I check my watch. The appointment was for eleven o'clock this morning and I got here at eleven on the dot. The minutes tick by. I'm getting more and more anxious the longer I wait. At quarter to twelve, I'm called into the doctor's office.

Dr. Williams is friendly and kind. "I know you've been waiting, Carlos. I apologize. It's been a busy morning here."

"That's OK." ***At least she said sorry***, I figure.

"Now let me pull up your file." She clicks on her computer keyboard for a minute. "I understand that you've been diagnosed with colorectal cancer, but the cancer has not yet spread to any nearby lymph nodes."

I pause and look at the stack of papers I've brought with me from my other doctor. I printed everything out. "Oh, uh, actually I think my doctor said it's spread to four lymph nodes already."

"Oh!" Dr. Williams's eyebrows raise in surprise as she squints at the computer screen, her mouth a thin line. "I apologize. You are correct. Our new IT system is a bit of a mess."

Is it a bad sign that the oncologist didn't know about the lymph nodes? My heart is racing, while my brain is buzzing with thoughts. ***And if this place has a bad IT system, what about the quality of the medicine they practice?***

I wish I'd asked my wife to come. I didn't want to worry her until I knew how serious this was. Now I have a million questions and no clue what to ask first. And English is my second language, so medical jargon or not, this is a lot. I can only fixate on one thing: ***Am I going to die?***

***

I can't believe I pulled up the wrong patient file. Our electronic health record (EHR) makes it hard to view information easily; I've complained about it before, and I'm especially annoyed by it now. Whether or not a cancer has spread to lymph nodes makes a big difference in the cancer's staging and subsequent treatment plan. I'm glad the patient spoke up.

I turn toward Carlos, making eye contact, and keeping my voice calm. He keeps fiddling with the papers in his hands and is clearly nervous. My heart goes out to him. I know that look of fear on his face; I see it all the time.

"So, with colorectal cancer, when it's spread to four to six nearby lymph nodes but not yet to distant sites, we classify it as stage IIIA."

"OK." He nods.

"At this point, the recommended course of treatment would be to remove the section of the colon where the cancer is present—a partial colectomy—along with the nearby lymph nodes, followed by adjuvant chemotherapy."

"OK," he says again. "Will I ... lose my hair?" he asks tentatively, before flushing red with embarrassment. "I'm sorry, that was a stupid question."

"No, it's not a stupid question at all!" I say quickly, at the same time surreptitiously glancing at the clock and seeing that I'm well behind in my appointments. But I can't end it here.

"Let's talk about your diagnosis and treatment options."

Thirty minutes later, we've talked through everything, and Carlos seems calmer. Still, as he leaves my office, there is a furrow of concern on his brow. As an oncologist, this is never easy—but before I know it, I'm on to the next patient, breaking more bad news. It's one of those days.

Best-selling author and thought leader Cy Wakeman suggests that accountability is "death to ego," explaining, "It's about one's belief as to whether or not they can have impact over their own outcomes and results."[20] In other words, a person cannot make another person accountable, but they can communicate expectations and related rewards and consequences. The choice to be accountable is individual. In this book, accountability is defined as follows:

Accountability: A commitment to performing the roles and responsibilities of a member of the team and fostering trust and respect, with the goal of supporting individuals to achieve the optimal patient-desired outcomes.

In this chapter's scenario, accountability is exercised by both Carlos and Dr. Williams, but with gaps resulting from the failures in communication. Carlos commits himself to what most individuals believe is expected of them as a patient—he shows up on time, he brings his paperwork, and he has his insurance information with him. Meanwhile, Dr. Williams likewise takes accountability, apologizing for the delay and acknowledging her mistake when she incorrectly references another patient's file.

Unfortunately, some members of the team don't show up ready to play. The receptionist is unfriendly. She takes no accountability for comfort or reassurance. As the first point of contact, this negatively impacts Carlos's confidence for upcoming stops in his healthcare journey. Next, an obsolete and difficult EHR is a root cause of Dr. Williams's delay in the clinical workflow, and is also an added risk—and a potential burnout factor. Finally, a lack of transparency and preparation for the real and possible costs, and of a full discussion of financial assistance and options, are both an insurance and healthcare system miss. The need to consider *all* touchpoints and team players in the patient journey becomes apparent, with both gaps and opportunities magnified.

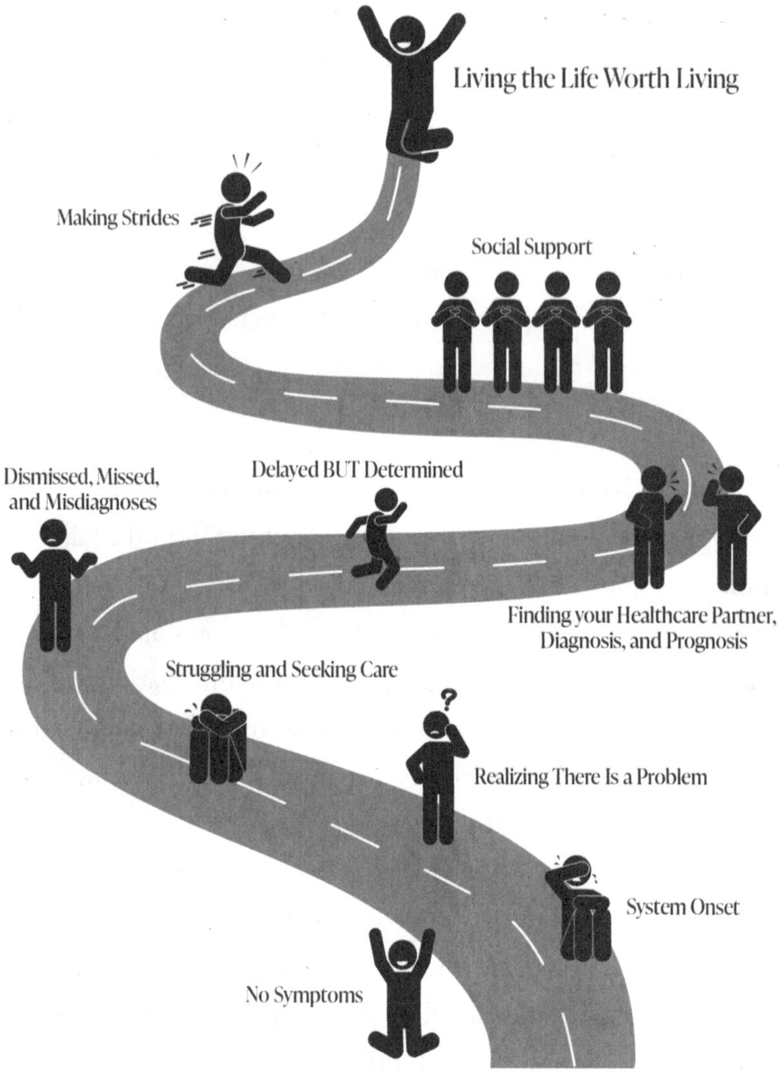

Figure 2.1: An illustration of the patient journey and its many touchpoints.

Communication failure further derails the misguided course for Carlos and Dr. Williams. Carlos is overwhelmed and scared—understandably. He wishes he had someone with him for support, such as his wife. English is his second language, so some of what is being discussed may not be clear to him. And his focus point—a fear of dying—is never communicated. While the deterrents for communicating his concerns are real, this failure to communicate results in a failure to rescue the misdirected relationship being built with his HCP and, worse, is potentially dangerous for his health.

Dr. Williams has a difficult and life-altering diagnosis to discuss while trying to function under suboptimal conditions: running behind schedule and experiencing EHR issues that result in her initially misstating important information. This impedes her ability to express the empathy she feels for Carlos. Although her apologetic response is socially appropriate, it does not help Carlos process his diagnosis. Instead, it could be useful to provide resources such as patient-friendly pamphlets and advocacy websites, especially those with Spanish translations.

Good intentions are not always reflective of optimal communication and accountability. In fact, research has found a discrepancy between the presumption of providers delivering compassionate care and patients actually receiving that same level of service. One survey showed that 75 percent of healthcare providers believed they did offer compassionate care, while just over 50 percent of patient respondents agreed with that.[21] Twenty-five percent of people reported leaving an appointment thinking something was missing, many without communicating that concern.

Clearly this is a setup for less-than-optimal satisfaction. There is a good chance Carlos will look for another oncologist, and Dr. Williams may become the face of failure in Carlos's eyes. Communication is the keystone, and when it fails, everything else falls apart. Carlos isn't failed by Dr. Williams specifically, but by the failure of the broader healthcare team and system. Without Carlos advocating for himself, this failure goes unchecked.

You Can't Control Everything

There is daily exposure to numerous factors that we can't control. These are things that fall into what researcher and author Stephen Covey calls the Circle of Concern. This is starkly contrasted by what we can control, or the Circle of Influence™, a term popularized by Covey and trademarked by Franklin Covey Co. Critical to this is concept is the individual control we have over our behavior, emotional response, and attitude in general—a superpower that each of us can continuously improve.

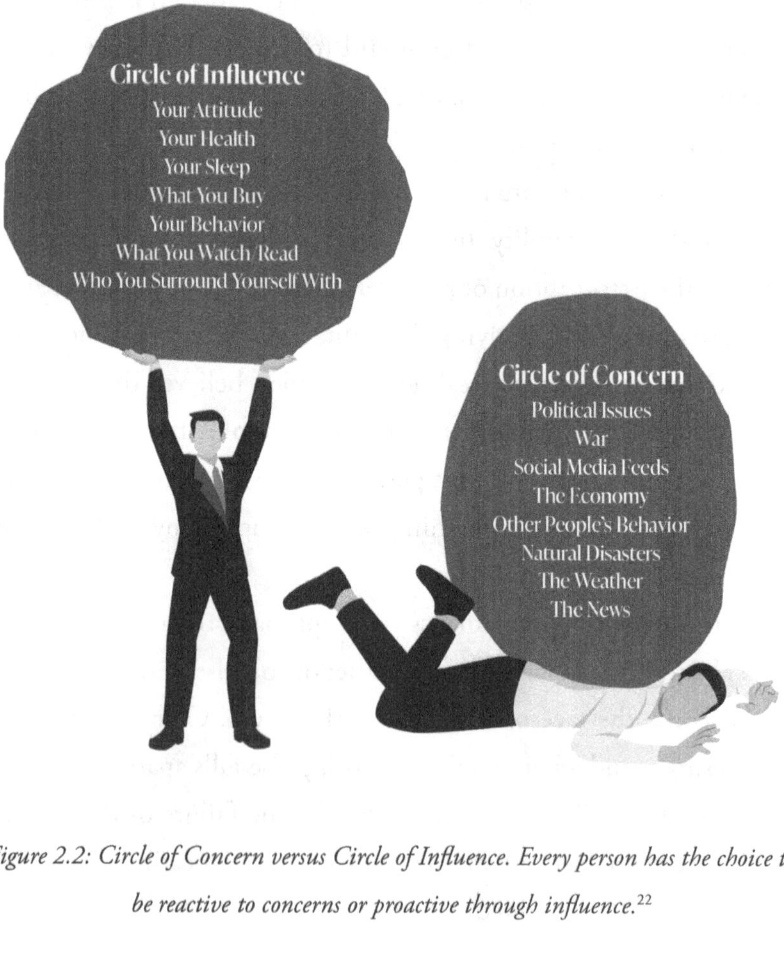

Figure 2.2: Circle of Concern versus Circle of Influence. Every person has the choice to be reactive to concerns or proactive through influence.[22]

Whether you're navigating your own medical journey or you're a member of the healthcare ecosystem, identify and utilize what you can control. You can't change the fact that you have been diagnosed with cancer, but you can control how you respond, who you surround yourself with, and how aggressive a treatment plan you pursue. Similarly, if you are a nurse or a doctor, you can't change the cancer diagnosis for your patient, but you can act with empathy, evaluate the patient's understanding, provide resources, and engage other team members to reduce barriers to care and optimize outcomes.

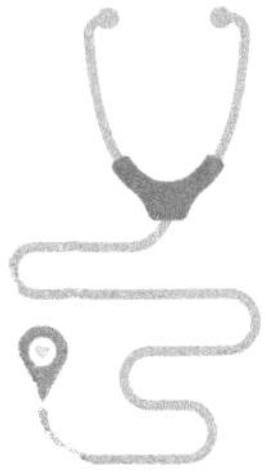

Communication Callout: Language Barriers

Language barriers can impede communication, resulting in reduced access, increased costs, dissatisfaction, and poorer quality care. For instance, limited English language proficiency (LELP) has been shown to increase the risk of being uninsured two- to fivefold, and further decreases the likelihood of having a usual HCP compared to primary English speakers.[23] LELP often results in delayed access to care and negatively impacts the relationship between the individual and the HCP.[24] This builds on prior research showcasing the consequences of poor communication, with almost 50 percent of participants with LELP experiencing an adverse event or harm as a result of impaired communication.[25] Proactive establishment of a patient's preferred spoken and read language, access to on-demand translation tools, and culturally sensitive preferred language resources can minimize barriers, reduce risks, and enhance comfort and confidence.

Exercising your ability to recognize and grow your sphere of control enhances your EQ and protects against the detriments of things that feel out of your control—which can be especially damaging to your confidence in and relationship with yourself. In medicine, burnout is real, with increasing numbers of professionals leaving or considering leaving clinical practice. The Physicians Foundation notes a 20 percent increase in the number of physicians reporting burnout, growing from 40 percent in 2018 to 60 percent in 2023.[26] Alarmingly, 70 percent of medical students also express feelings of burnout. Recognizing what you can control reduces feelings of frustration and vulnerability and minimizes the risk of potential disability.

The risk of physician burnout becomes clearer when considering the shift to VBO. This model exclusively holds providers accountable for improving patient outcomes by measuring the quality of healthcare and patient outcomes in relation to the cost of care. Say a person with obesity, high blood pressure, diabetes, and obstructive sleep apnea has a clinical visit with an endocrinologist for poorly controlled diabetes. After careful evaluation, education, and discussion with the patient about the best course of treatment, the specialist does the following: sends a prescription to the pharmacy; orders additional follow-up labs; gives the patient referrals to a diabetes educator, a weight management specialist, and a nutritionist; and schedules a follow-up for six weeks' time.

The following day, the patient goes to the pharmacy to get their prescription filled. However, the patient's insurance states that the drug is not on formulary: an alternative must be prescribed, or the doctor will need to contact the patient's insurance company and provide medical necessity documentation. The patient calls and leaves a message for the doctor's office. The following day, the patient receives a callback stating that the doctor has sent a letter of medical necessity but that the insurance can take up to seventy-two hours to review and respond to the request (and can still deny it). A day later, the insurance approves the medication, but this information is not communicated to the patient. Two weeks go by, and the patient still hasn't gotten any medication.

At the follow-up appointment six weeks later, there has been *some* improvement in the patient's results, thanks to the lifestyle changes he has implemented. But the review of his daily blood glucose demonstrates he is still far from his goal. The doctor apologizes when the patient explains that he didn't know the medication had been approved and encourages him to pick it up that day. However, the patient is now six weeks behind in his treatment and has reduced confidence in the system. His mounting frustration impedes the likelihood of persistence with the plan.

In this model, the failures of communication on the side of the insurance and the pharmacy are not met with consequences. Their lack of accountability negatively impacts the patient's outcome—and, consequently, the VBO determination of the specialist. This kind of model puts an even greater strain on already overburdened HCPs. The scenario also shows how access to care is obstructed by a greater lack of accountability in the healthcare system—a system where the focus is often on minimizing cost, not mitigating risk.

Healthcare Is a Team Effort

Unfortunately, historical and current environments still emphasize the clinician as the gatekeeper of best outcomes. Although medicine has moved from a paternalistic model of care delivery (in which an HCP makes decisions for a patient) to a shared care decision-making model (in which HCPs and patients work together to determine the course of care), I would advocate for an even more radical option: a patient- (person-)directed model of care that abandons episodic transactional care and replaces it with a longitudinal model of continuous care delivery using both synchronous and asynchronous methods. Empower the patient. Give them the steering wheel to drive toward the desired destination with their HCP as the GPS—and with the support of others within the healthcare ecosystem to avoid the potholes, unnecessary detours, and near misses.

Healthcare isn't an individual sport. There is a whole team of individuals and organizations, each playing a part and influencing the others. We might picture it like a stacked Venn diagram where everything is built around the needs and support of the patient, with each contributor layering on additional shared resources and responsibilities for success:

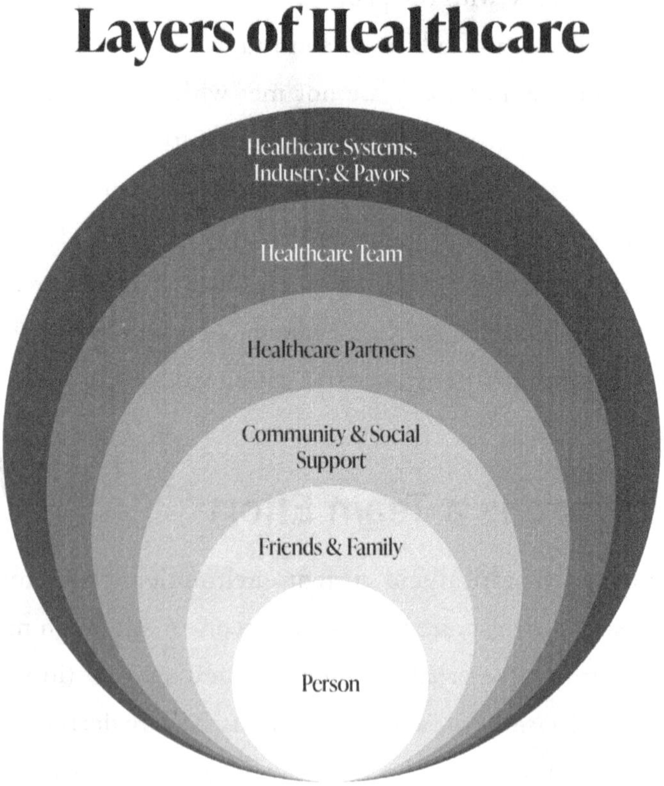

Figure 2.1: Healthcare as a team effort comprised of multiple layers.

Following this model, you have different people, organizations, and systems accountable for the different pieces of the healthcare journey. Let's look at some of the considerations, focusing on the factors that each player in the ecosystem can control.

The patient can control:

- **Availability:** Do they take the time for appointments and follow-ups?
- **Preparedness:** Do they bring the documentation they need, such as past medical records?
- **Communication needs:** Do they have any communication needs they should flag? For example, do they need an interpreter? Are they prepared to ask questions when something is unclear? Are they aware of their own health literacy limitations?

The HCP and healthcare support team can control:

- **Availability:** Is the HCP team available in different ways—say, on site versus telemedicine? Can they accommodate diverse patient schedules; for example, by opening early for before-work appointments?
- **Scheduling:** Is scheduling appointments easy? What tools can patients use to schedule? Are front-desk staff required to juggle calls, texts, emails, and online scheduling tools? Is the system streamlined?
- **Triage system:** What order are patients treated in? When do they need to be sent on for emergency care? If they're in the ER, how long will they need to wait?

- **Workflows and care pathways:** Is there a clear workflow and care pathway in place? If a patient comes in with X complaint, what's the Y step to take?
- **Relationships with other staff:** Is the healthcare workplace a positive environment? Is collaboration prioritized over competition? Are more experienced individuals providing training and mentorship? Research has shown that communication is improved when there is a team consideration in healthcare, such as faculty supporting residents.[27]
- **Established referral networks and ease of use:** If the physician refers the patient to a specialist, what process ensues? Does the patient have to find someone, or is there a direct referral process?
- **Communication tools:** Does the healthcare team use diverse communication tools? What about educational materials? What about visuals, such as graphics and videos?

Communication Callout: Health Literacy

Health literacy refers to a person's ability to find, understand, and use information and services to support health-related decision-making for themselves. Patients with low health literacy may benefit from different educational formats, such as graphics instead of written text. Patients have a responsibility to recognize their own limitations in terms of health literacy, while HCPs, healthcare support teams, and other system players—such as patient groups—have a responsibility to deliver multimodal educational tools for patients.

Then, there are the components that patients, HCPs, and healthcare support teams have less control over—these are more systemic:

- **Access:** What healthcare options are available to a patient—geographically, logistically, and financially?
- **Social support:** Does the patient have family, friends, and other pillars of support to accompany them on their healthcare journey? Are there external sources of support, such as peer mentors?
- **Patient resources:** What disease-specific resources, about topics including diagnosis, testing, treatments, and side effects, are available? Patient groups can be valuable.
- **Diversity resources:** Is the ecosystem mindful about how different types of individuals are approached? Are HCPs and patients harnessing these resources? Are diversity, equity, and inclusion measures lived, or are they just given lip service?
- **Non-medical supports:** A healthcare condition can impact everything from whether a person can work to whether they can complete activities of daily living. Examples of non-medical supports could include transport services or meal prep programs.

How many of the points above can you control? Definitely not all of them. I don't want that to be disheartening! Rather, I hope that realization empowers you to take a firmer hold on what you *can* control—while also realizing that the accountability doesn't fall solely on you.

A NARRATIVE CASE STUDY, REIMAGINED

Our narrative case study of Carlos and Dr. Williams is one example of the difference a team approach to accountability can make. What if the exchange we saw in the introduction had taken that mindset into account?

I'm terrified. Stage three colon cancer. Does this mean I'm going to die? My mouth is dry as I approach the reception desk at the doctor's office.

"It's going to be fine," my wife, Elena, says, squeezing my hand. She has a plastic folder of papers in her other hand—my health records.

"Good morning! How can I help?" The girl behind the front desk greets us cheerfully.

"Good morning. I have an appointment with Dr. Williams." I slide my insurance card across the desk.

"Great!" She picks up the card and checks my name. "Mr. Ruiz. I can get you checked in down here, but note that oncology is on the fourth floor. The elevators are just behind you, to the right."

"Got it." I nod.

"I'm afraid we are running behind today, so there may be a bit of a wait ... I am sorry about that." She looks apologetic. "We do have free Wi-Fi, so feel free to connect to that. The passwords are posted in the waiting room." She takes my insurance information and sends us on our way.

Twenty minutes later, we're upstairs, waiting to be called into the doctor's office. My appointment was for eleven o'clock this morning, but it's quarter to twelve by the time we're called in. I aimlessly scroll on social media while we wait.

Dr. Williams is kind. "I know you've been waiting, Carlos. I apologize. It's been a busy morning."

"That's OK." ***At least she said sorry,*** I figure. "This is my wife, Elena."

"Very nice to meet you both. Now, let me just pull up your file." She clicks on her computer keyboard for a minute before looking back to us. "I understand that you've been diagnosed with colorectal cancer and that it's spread to four lymph nodes already."

My wife is already looking at the paperwork in her hands. "Yes, that's what they told us." I nod, reassured that the doctor is familiar with my case.

"OK, so you probably have some questions about what that means exactly."

Elena and I exchange glances. I nod. ***Yes.*** The biggest question: ***Am I going to die?***

***

I take another look at Carlos's file, which I've pulled up on my computer screen. I'm glad our new IT system is working; everything is clearly organized. Then, I turn toward Carlos, making eye contact and keeping my voice calm. His wife has one hand over his, and I'm glad he brought a family member to support him.

I start the explanation. "So, with colorectal cancer, when it's spread to four to six nearby lymph nodes but not yet to distant sites, we'd classify it as stage IIIA."

"OK." Carlos nods.

"And what does IIIA mean exactly?" his wife cuts in. "Is that ... treatable?" The pause over the word ***treatable*** is slight but there. I know what she's asking me. ***Is he going to be OK?***

"Elena, this is an important question. Very commonly, the question that many people who are diagnosed with cancer will ask is about prognosis. Is this treatable? Will I die? I am purposefully sharing what I have heard from others who have been in your position because, in the past, they have often had trouble asking those questions—even though they were the ones they wanted answers to most. Would it be helpful for me to discuss the answers to those questions with you now?"

Carlos and his wife look back at me and, in harmony, respond with a timid "Yes."

So, I get into it: the details of the diagnosis; the additional testing needed to get more information about the cancer; the factors of Carlos's personal and family health history that are favorable or concerning; what has been studied in this stage of cancer, along with the different treatment options; clinical trials that are occurring that may or may not be considered ... I provide an overarching understanding of the cancer in general, but tailored to Carlos's circumstances, making sure to use visuals to demonstrate key points.

I pause. "That was a lot of information, so I want to pause and ask what questions you have. Is there anything I can answer for you right now?" Both shake their heads ***no***. "Should I proceed with discussing next steps?" I ask. Both nod *yes*.

Thirty minutes later, we've talked through a lot—but I have no doubt they still have questions. I send them off with some pamphlets and tips for online resources that can provide more information and support. After Carlos mentions that his native language is Spanish, I make sure to point him toward Spanish-language resources. I want him to be comfortable with the information he's receiving.

In this scenario, the difference a team approach can make becomes clear. First, Carlos has his wife with him. As he is overwhelmed by information and worried about his health, having someone else by his side to ask questions and confirm information can help him better understand his situation and feel supported.

Next, consider the entry into the building. Carlos is greeted warmly and clearly directed to where he needs to go. The receptionist is up front and apologetic about the wait. Greater consideration is shown than in the first scenario.

The doctor's experience with the patient file points to another key player in the healthcare team, a behind-the-scenes player—the EHR. In the opening scenario, Dr. Williams struggled with a clunky EHR system. In this scenario, the EHR system is easy to operate, and the doctor can quickly pull up Carlos's file without errors. Carlos gains confidence, as he sees that his doctor knows his case.

As in the previous scenario, Dr. Williams takes the time to explain the diagnosis and treatment options. However, this time, the doctor doesn't just wait for potential questions but infers what Carlos and Elena may be wondering and worrying about—those scary unspoken questions regarding prognosis.

Finally, the doctor uses not only words but also visual aids when explaining the facts. And, lastly, Dr. Williams sends Carlos and Elena off with additional information, from reputable, physician-approved resources—including some in Carlos's native language.

Which encounter do you think leaves the patient feeling comforted—and the doctor feeling confident? This is what happens when the whole team comes together to create the conditions for shared accountability.

COMMUNITY SUPPORT

Cancer is a complex illness that takes a huge toll on patients and their families. Treatment can also be costly, with many patients going into debt.[28] Given the complexity, it's essential that patients can access resources addressing the varied implications. Excellent sources of knowledge have been produced by the **American Cancer Society**, the **National Cancer Institute**, and the **National Comprehensive Cancer Network**. Links to each of these are included in Appendix B.

Having a strong support team is essential when facing something as scary as a cancer diagnosis. With an understanding of their personal circles of influence, patients, HCPs, and healthcare support teams can articulate accountability while protecting time and effort. As the patient's journey continues, that team effort must be maintained. The next step? The meet-and-greet.

Growth Opportunity: Proactive, Not Reactive, Mindset

Consider your role in the healthcare ecosystem. What can *you* control? For example, if you're an HCP, you can control how you convey information. If you're a person on your own healthcare journey or a caregiver or support for a patient, you can share openly with your HCP, schedule and maintain your appointments, relay new information or concerns if they arise, and ask questions when you don't understand something.

Irrespective of your role in the healthcare journey, try this exercise to establish a proactive mindset:

1. Make a list of your goals.

2. Define what resources or support are needed, if any, to get to those goals.

3. Note what barriers exist to meeting the goals.

Now go through each of the needs and barriers and identify what you can influence and how. This is your road map to taking control of what you can. The QR code links to additional resources to help.

Chapter 2 Endnotes

20 Cy Wakeman, "Redefining Accountability in the Workplace," *Medium*, March 26, 2017, https://medium.com/@CyWakeman/redefining-accountability-in-the-workplace-1e880b4246d6.

21 Beth A. Lown, Julie Rosen, and John Marttila, "An Agenda for Improving Compassionate Care: A Survey Shows About Half of Patients Say Such Care is Missing," *Health Affairs (Millwood)* 30, no. 9 (2011): 1772–8, https://doi.org/10.1377/hlthaff.2011.0539.

22 Stephen R. Covey, *The 7 Habits of Highly Effective People: Powerful Lessons in Personal Change*, anniversary edition (Simon & Schuster, 2013).

23 Andriana M. Foiles Sifuentes, Monica Robledo Cornejo, Nien Chen Li, Maira A. Castaneda-Avila, Jennifer Tjia, and Kate L. Lapane, "The Role of Limited English Proficiency and Access to Health Insurance and Health Care in the Affordable Care Act Era," *Health Equity* 4, no. 1 (2020): 509–517, https://doi.org/10.1089/heq.2020.0057.

24 Mamata Pandey, R. Geoffrey Maina, Jonathan Amoyaw, Yiyan Li, Rejina Kamrul, C. Rocha Michaels et al., "Impacts of English Language Proficiency on Healthcare Access, Use, and Outcomes Among Immigrants: A Qualitative Study," *BMC Health Services Research* 21, no. 741 (2021): 1–13, https://doi.org/10.1186/s12913-021-06750-4.

25 Chandrika Divi, Richard G. Koss, Stephen P. Schmaltz, and Jerod M. Loeb, "Language Proficiency and Adverse Events in US Hospitals: A Pilot Study," *Journal of the International Society for Quality in Health Care* 19, no. 2 (2007): 60–67, https://doi.org/10.1093/intqhc/mzl069.

26 "Taking the Pulse on Physicians to Spur Action," The Physicians Foundation, accessed December 4, 2024, https://physiciansfoundation.org/surveys/.

27 Caroline E. Rassbach, Alyssa L. Bogetz, Nicola Orlov, Alisa McQueen, Vasudah Bhavaraju, David Mahoney et al., "The Effect of Faculty Coaching on Resident Attitudes, Confidence, and Patient-Rated Communication: A Multi-Institutional Randomized Controlled Trial," *Academic Pediatrics* 19, no. 2 (2018): 186–194, https://doi.org/10.1016/j.acap.2018.10.004.

28 Noam N. Levey, "In America, Cancer Patients Endure Debt on Top of Disease," *KFF Health News*, July 9, 2022, https://kffhealthnews.org/news/article/in-america-cancer-patients-endure-debt-on-top-of-disease/.

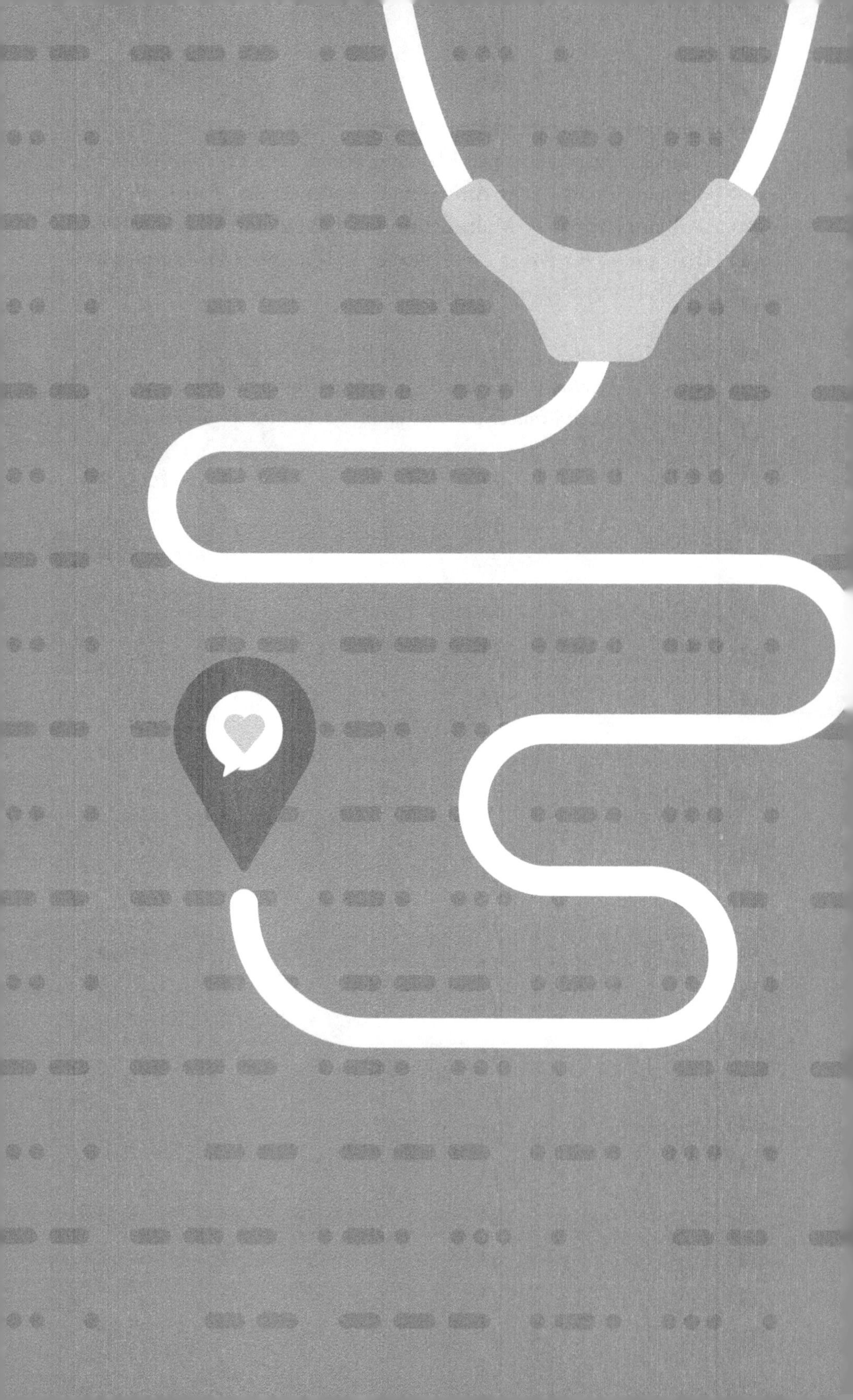

CHAPTER 3

The Meet-and-Greet

The purpose of this chapter is to build on the proactive mindset and set the stage for the pivotal first meeting between the HCP and the patient. The foundation of a successful relationship and the achievement of optimal outcomes is predicated on starting off with transparent bidirectional communication that will feed the development of trust, respect, and collaboration.

NARRATIVE CASE STUDY: A PATIENT WITH OBESITY STRUGGLES WITH KNEE PAIN

Omar is seeing Dr. Greene for the first time. Omar has struggled with his weight for years and is actively trying to shed pounds. However, today, he's seeing Dr. Greene for a very specific, unrelated reason—his knee pain.

"Nice to meet you, Dr. Greene." I limp into the doctor's room, trying not to wince with each step.

"Nice to meet you, too, Omar. Please, take a seat." I'm so used to people just calling me "O" that I almost ask *who?!* when I hear my given first name. The doctor gives me a quick glance, up and down, before looking back at his computer screen. "I see you're here for knee pain?"

Did he not see me limp in here like one of my legs is made of wood?

"Yeah, it's killing me, Doc!" I shake my head and give a nervous chuckle. The truth is, I am embarrassed about how this happened–while I was working out. "I've been noticing it after my workouts, but yesterday, after I was on the treadmill, it was really bad."

"Treadmill workouts lead to injury even in people who are very lean."

Wait, did my doctor just call me fat?

"I mean, I am trying to lose the weight."

"I'm glad to hear that. Obesity comes with a lot of issues, like hypertension and diabetes." Dr. Greene eyes me over his glasses. "Are you exercising regularly and eating a nutritious diet?"

"I try, but you know ... It's not perfect." *Did I* not *just tell him I'm trying?!*

"Mmm." Dr. Greene click-clacks on his keyboard for a second.

Man, this guy sucks. I almost wish I'd just popped an Advil and skipped the doctor altogether. I'm sure my knee will get better on its own anyway.

***

A look at Omar's medical file is quite concerning. His cholesterol is high. He's hypertensive. He's prediabetic. And he's not even forty! If he doesn't get his weight under control, none of this will improve. I really want to help this guy. What can I do to get him on track?

"Maybe working with a nutritionist would help," I suggest. "There are some local programs where you can get expert guidance through your insurance provider ..." My voice trails off as I squint at the computer screen, searching for the program I'm thinking of.

When I look back to Omar, I see that he's on his phone—apparently not paying any attention. I feel a flicker of annoyance, until Omar holds up his phone to show me the screen. ***Oh God, it's WebMD.*** "I was googling what might have happened to my knee, and it looks like it could be patellofemoral stress syndrome?"

"Knee pain can have many different causes, so we can't be sure just yet," I reply. "In any case, obesity can increase the risk of several causes of knee pain. But the good news is that we can change that."

I smile encouragingly at Omar. He is young enough to turn his health around. And I want to help him do just that.

A first impression can be the last impression, and, similar to accountability, one person's perception of an interaction can be divergent from the other's intentions. In this chapter's scenario, communication fails because both sides are coming from positions of differing priorities and perceptions, despite appropriate intent and shared concerns. Omar's perception of Dr. Greene is that he is fat-shaming him and dismissing his primary concern of knee pain. Meanwhile, Dr. Greene does not adequately convey why his concerns about Omar's weight are related to the reason for his visit—his knee pain—or that he is trying to take a whole-person approach to optimizing Omar's health.

Both parties try to convey their perspectives while failing to recognize that each other's priorities are related. Self-imposed barriers to observing and listening to one another interfere. Dr. Greene is perceived as distracted, as he diligently reviews Omar's record with mounting concern while not observing the limp and the non-verbal expression of pain. He greets Omar by his first name, despite reviewing the EHR that displays his preferred name as "O." And Dr. Greene's intention to "rescue" Omar from orthopedic and cardiometabolic consequence with a focus on weight management is received as ignoring Omar's primary concern—his knee pain.

In an attempt to redirect the focus to his own concern, O brings up a patient-facing resource (WebMD) that he thinks may accurately describe the cause of his knee pain. Unfortunately, his searching for this information is perceived as disinterest and just scrolling on his phone.

The reality is that both Omar and Dr. Greene *do* care. Intentions are lost in translation, replaced by individual priorities and perceptions that segregate efforts rather than facilitating partnership. Social awareness is complimentary to self-awareness (both discussed earlier, in the EQ paradigm).

Communication Callout: Explicit/Implicit Bias

Bias is a part of life, as much as we'd like to pretend it's not. Recognizing explicit bias can be easy. Implicit bias is a whole other animal. Although Dr. Greene may not realize it, in our scenario, he is showing bias toward Omar by assuming that the patient is not taking steps to care for himself and lose weight. The doctor recognizes that Omar is obese and makes this assumption, which, in turn, changes his approach to Omar's care. In healthcare, where life-altering decisions may be made, this is a huge problem. We must always recognize the presence of bias if we are going to challenge it.

There Is Only *One* First Impression

Irrespective of intention, poor perception can jeopardize the ability to successfully build a relationship based on trust, respect, and collaboration. In the healthcare context, the HCP is rarely the first point of contact. From front-desk staff to nurses, a person seeking care usually sees other people before they step into the physical or virtual exam room. Think of Carlos's interaction with the receptionist in the previous chapter—it wasn't pleasant. Those split seconds of interaction are important. Again, it's a team effort! If the first experience with the health system is bad, it may be perceived that the medical care is bad, too.

As in the previous scenarios, there are systemic issues that place a strain on the situation. Medical systems generally put pressure on HCPs to see more patients, more quickly. To a busy HCP with a waiting room full of people and an EHR inbox full of messages, test results, and other demands, efficiency feels critical to survival. Ten minutes of chitchat is an indulgence that seems impossible to afford. The good news? It doesn't take ten minutes to have a positive meet-and-greet—and there are things that both the patient and the HCP can do to make the most of the brief time they have together. Let's examine what is in your control during an appointment.

As the HCP, consider your appearance and demeanor. Competing priorities can make you feel disheveled, rushed, and even burned out, but it is a part of self-management to choose how you show up. Choose to have a put-together appearance, to take time to prepare and be present, and to lead with empathy and interest. If you are conducting telemedicine appointments, consider your surrounding environment as a part of your appearance. When reviewing the patient's chart, ensure you are informed on their preferred name and who else may be accompanying them in the room to ensure an appropriate introduction.

As the person seeking care, formulate an idea of what the goal of your visit is. Using a symptom diary can help you identify your goal for the visit and provide important information to help identify next steps (later chapters will provide more details on symptom diaries, including a template). Bring copies or access details to any information you may have collected previously that may be relevant to the visit (test results, consult notes, referral requests). For a telemedicine appointment, ensure you are in a location that is quiet and safe and which allows for you to speak freely without concerns about compromising your privacy. If you have others with you, provide an introduction of who they are and what your expectation of their role may be, as well as any limitations on how you want them to participate.

Communication Callout: Telemedicine

Virtual meet-and-greets are becoming increasingly common, as they are convenient without compromising the quality of care. For phone or video calls, ensure you connect in a location that has good reception or Wi-Fi to avoid disruption. Put away other distractions. Finally, if you are looking at something else on your screen during the call, address it by saying something like, "I'm just looking at your patient file on the screen here." The other person can tell when you are reading or looking at something else, and you don't want them to assume you aren't tuned in.

A successful meet-and-greet starts with both sides participating and setting expectations for each step. As an HCP, start with a simple empathetic statement summarizing your understanding of the patient's chief complaint, their motivating reason for the appointment. This can be followed by any observations and then a confirmatory question such as, "Is this accurate?" This question allows for the correction of any errors in understanding and reinforces a partnership. For example: "Mr. Johnson, my understanding is that the reason you are here is for right knee pain. I observed you limping when you walked in. I am sorry you are in pain. Is this accurate, or is there anything else you are hoping to cover today?"

As the person seeking care, the meet-and-greet is also an opportunity to advocate for yourself and ensure that you are confirming your intention for the visit. Share concerns regarding any challenges or misdirection that may be negatively influencing your comfort, perception, or experience. Make your HCP aware of these and allow them to respond. In chapter 9, we will examine strategies that can be implemented to help redirect and rebuild fractured relationships.

Frameworks for Successful First Impressions

There are a few frameworks that HCPs and their supporting teams can use to create good first impressions. For instance, research has shown a positive impact on patient experiences and satisfaction at a medical practice when the front-desk staff are trained in AIDET™ communication.[29] AIDET stands for the following:

- **Acknowledge:** Acknowledge the patient, making eye contact and greeting them by their name. Acknowledge family or friends in the room.
- **Introduce:** Introduce yourself with your name, professional certification, and experience.
- **Duration:** Give a time expectation for the physician's arrival and any test results. Identify next steps. If no estimate can be given, let the patient know when you'll update them.
- **Explanation:** Explain step-by-step what to expect and answer questions. Let the patient know how to reach you (for example, with a nurse call button).
- **Thank you:** Thank the patient and accompanying family/friends.

AIDET has been shown to reduce patient anxiety in nursing settings.[30] Research posits that AIDET, combined with a "Commit to Sit" policy (taking the time to take a seat, rather than remaining standing) and care for cultural competency, can improve the overall quality of patient-centered care.[31] And medical residents who underwent skills training in AIDET showed a significant improvement in communication value.[32] AIDET can be adapted for various roles, from front-desk to nursing staff.

Another model is the C-I-CARE strategy. C-I-CARE is a framework used to structure best practice communications and develop relationship-based care approaches with patients, families, and colleagues. C-I-CARE stands for:

- **C**onnect with people by calling them by their preferred names.
- **I**ntroduce yourself.
- **C**ommunicate what you're going to do and why.
- **A**sk permission before every action.
- **R**espond to patient questions or requests promptly.
- **E**xit courteously and always with an explanation of what will come next.

At the meet-and-greet stage, the first two points are relevant—connect and introduce. The other points will become relevant in later stages, such as history-taking and exam time (and we will cover those in upcoming chapters). Like AIDET, C-I-CARE has shown benefits—for example, in minimizing the risk of post-intensive care syndrome (PICS). PICS is a term used to describe a constellation of new or worsened dysfunctions in critically ill patients after their discharge from the intensive care unit (ICU). A study showed that, when combined with positive motivational psychological interventions, C-I-CARE communication in nursing may have a positive effect in relieving PICS.[33]

Patients also have a role to play. Steps patients can take to make sure they are heard include:

- **Setting expectations:** What do you hope to get from the appointment?
- **Making time:** Arrive early to take care of admin before you see the physician.
- **Preparing your paperwork:** Although this goes beyond the meet-and-greet to later stages of the interaction, it's worth mentioning here. Do you have your medical files, referrals, insurance details, symptom diary, and anything else that's relevant?
- **Being ready to advocate for yourself:** Prepare to advocate for yourself, whether it's a matter of requesting language assistance or asserting what name you like to be called by.
- **Tuning in:** Dial in to the interaction! Put your phone in your bag or pocket; if it's in your hand, it can be tempting to play with it.

Successfully reaching the destination in a healthcare journey requires EQ, buy-in, and accountability on both sides. Securing that buy-in starts with the meet-and-greet. As an HCP, if you fail in the meet-and-greet, you risk the patient not communicating transparently with you. That's not to say it's all on the physician's side! If you are on your medical journey, be proactive and convey your concerns clearly, and advocate for yourself when necessary.

Whatever the medium, whether it's face-to-face or digital, give the meet-and-greet the attention it deserves. This is the first and potentially *only* opportunity to establish respect and trust. Make it count!

A NARRATIVE CASE STUDY, REIMAGINED

How might Omar and Dr. Greene's interaction have changed if each had given more care to the meet-and-greet? Let's see.

"Nice to meet you, Dr. Greene." I limp into the doctor's room, trying not to wince with each step. I usually have my phone glued to my hand, but I've put it in my pocket now.

"Nice to meet you, too, Mr. Woods." The doctor stands up to greet me. "Is Mr. Woods OK, or do you prefer I call you something else?"

"Just 'O' is cool." I take the seat the doctor points to. His eyes are on me the whole time, and he has a nice smile.

"It looks like you might be favoring your left leg when you walk, O. Am I seeing that right?"

"Yes, it's killing me!"

"I understand that's why you're here?"

"Yes, sir."

"OK, I'm just going to take a look at your file. Give me just one moment, please ..." The doctor pauses to look at his computer screen. "So, you're here for knee pain. I guess we already figured that out. Do you know when it started?"

I tell him I've been noticing knee pain after my workouts. Before I know it, Dr. Greene is asking me one question after the next about my knee, my workouts, my diet—all kinds of stuff! I thought he'd just take a look at my knee and order me an x-ray or something, but he's full of questions. He seems chill, though, so I don't mind answering them.

I also feel comfortable telling him I've already done some research. "I googled my symptoms, and I read about something called—hang on, it's on my phone." I pull it out and look at the screen. "Patellofemoral stress syndrome?" I feel kind of embarrassed admitting this—I'm probably way off—but Dr. Greene just nods.

"Actually, if you've been doing your treadmill workouts on an incline, that's not unfeasible. Have you?"

***

"Yeah, I have," O confirms, his face lighting up, when I ask him if he's been walking on the treadmill on an incline.

"We need to take a look before we can confirm anything, but it's a possibility." Sometimes Dr. Google can be helpful. I'm eager to figure out what's going on with O's knee—but looking at his medical records, there are some other things I want to discuss, too.

"O, I'm looking at your file, and there are some other things I do want to talk about other than the knee pain. Your cholesterol is high, and your blood sugar is also higher than ideal."

"Yeah, that's why I was working out in the first place. I'm trying to lose some weight."

This is great news—it's every doctor's dream. A patient who is already aware of the problem and is trying to change. Now, what can I do to help him succeed?

"Maybe we can look at some workouts that put less stress on your joints." I reach for the pamphlet I have on low-impact exercises to send him home with. "And there are some programs I know of that might be able to help you with your diet, too."

"That sounds good." O smiles.

"Good! But first, let's take a closer look at what's going on with that knee."

The content of this conversation is pretty much the same as what we saw in the first version of the interaction: weight management and knee pain. However, the exchange has a much more productive outcome, largely because of how it starts. In those first seconds, Dr. Greene shows interest and respect—and while he addresses Omar's weight, he doesn't dismiss the reason Omar is there today: his knee pain.

The groundwork has been set for a productive partnership. It seems likely that Dr. Greene will continue to accompany Omar on his wellness journey. This is the kind of healthcare partnership that can result in better outcomes in the big picture, not just in this one instance of joint pain.

COMMUNITY SUPPORT

Most American adults struggle with being overweight—yet there's still a lot of stigma around the topic, which can influence an everyday meet-and-greet. Data shows that 75 percent of American adults struggle with being overweight, and of those, 42 percent have obesity.[34] Unfortunately, stigma often paints the picture that affected individuals don't care, aren't trying to lose weight, or are making a choice to remain overweight. Such stigma can negatively impact a medical journey. HCPs must recognize bias, while patients must prepare to advocate for themselves. Gain an understanding of how being overweight can impact your health, recognize signs of related concerns, and research ways to advocate for yourself. The **Centers for Disease Control and Prevention**, the **American Society for Nutrition**, and the **Obesity Action Coalition** have resources to help, which I've linked to in Appendix B.

The meet-and-greet between an HCP and a patient can take less than sixty seconds. While that first impression is critical, the need for attentive, focused communication doesn't stop there. With trust established, it's time to take the patient's history.

Growth Opportunity: Your Meet-and-Greet Checklist

How you prepare for the meet-and-greet will depend on your role in the healthcare ecosystem. A quick checklist can help you prepare for making that positive first impression, whatever your role may be. Scan the QR code to access one checklist for support staff, one for patients, and one for HCPs.

Chapter 3 Endnotes

29 Thien T. Nguyen, "The Effect of AIDET Communications Delivered by Front Desk Staff on Patient Experience and Satisfaction at a Medical Practice" (doctorate thesis, Capella University, 2019), ProQuest Dissertations & Theses (13427293), https://www.proquest.com/openview/c584ec9cbf93119b13f345931407bafb.

30 Kun Fu, Shuping Li, and Sufen Lu, "Application and Effect Evaluation on Acknowledge-Introduce-Duration-Explanation-Thank You (AIDET) Communication Mode in Cataract Daytime Operation Nursing," *Annals of Eye Science* 5 (June 2020), https://doi.org/10.21037/aes.2020.03.01.

31 Tiffany Nguyen, "Implementing AIDET and Commit to Sit to Increase Patient Satisfaction in the Pediatric Outpatient Setting" (master's thesis, University of San Francisco, 2022), University of San Francisco Master's Projects and Capstones (1365), https://repository.usfca.edu/capstone/1365.

32 Andrea Mechanick Braverman, Elisabeth J. Kunkel, Leo Katz, Austin Katona, Theresa Heavens, Andrew Miller et al., "Do I Buy It? How AIDET™ Training Changes Residents' Values About Patient Care," *Journal of Patient Experience* 2, no. 1 (2015): 13–20, https://doi.org/10.1177/237437431500200104.

33 Sun-Ju She and Ying-Ying Xu, "Effect of CICARE Communication Nursing Model Combined with Motivational Psychological Intervention in Patients with Post-Intensive Care Unit Syndrome," *World Journal of Psychiatry* 13, no. 9 (2019): 707–713, https://doi.org/10.5498/wjp.v13.i9.707.

34 "Overweight & Obesity Statistics," National Institute of Diabetes and Digestive and Kidney Diseases, accessed December 4, 2024, https://www.niddk.nih.gov/health-information/health-statistics/overweight-obesity.

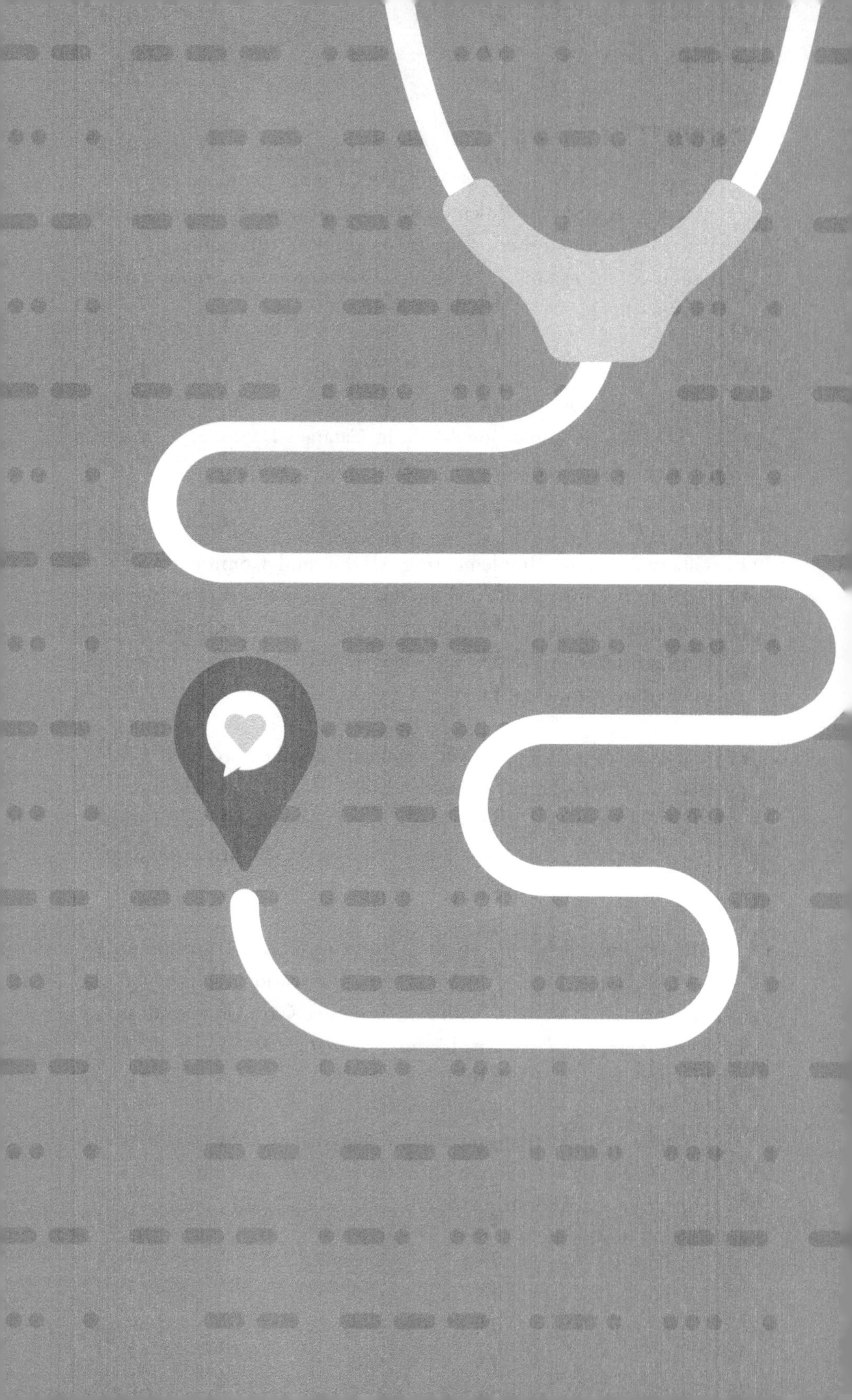

CHAPTER 4

Everyone Has History/ Her-Story/Their-Story

The purpose of this chapter is to guide logical, objective history-sharing/taking, while also emphasizing that history-sharing is *always* subjective. As noted in chapter 3, personal perceptions, biases, and contexts can impact relationship building. This makes the need for focused, intentional information gathering all the more important.

NARRATIVE CASE STUDY: A MIGRAINE SUFFERER SEEKS RELIEF

Michelle is looking to Dr. Pearson for help with migraines, which she's been experiencing for six months. She's nineteen, making this one of her first "adult" doctor appointments without her mom present.

Ugh. These fluorescent lights are terrible. I squint into the blaring whiteness of the doctor's office. This light sensitivity probably means I have a migraine coming on. Great.

"So, now that we've got the introductions out of the way, I'd like to ask you some questions about your migraines," Dr. Pearson says in his booming voice. I have to stop myself from wincing at the sound.

"Sure." I try to concentrate as he starts firing off an endless list of questions.

"How much do you sleep at night?"

"Uh, six hours, maybe? Seven?"

"When was your last migraine?"

"Last week," I reply confidently.

"Day? Night?"

"Uh, it started creeping up on me in the morning, I think?" I'm not sure.

"And how long did it last?"

"Maybe five hours?" I have no clue. When my head is throbbing, time stands still.

"Did you have any other symptoms accompanying the migraine?"

"Symptoms?"

"Like nausea, vomiting, light sensitivity ..."

"Yes! Light sensitivity."

"And do you drink or smoke?"

I pause. I'm not twenty-one!

"Please be honest, Michelle. I'm not here to judge." Dr. Pearson gives me a smile. But I feel like I'm talking to my dad. Admitting that I technically break the law by drinking underage feels weird.

"Yeah, I have a beer now and then with friends. And I smoke when I drink."

"OK, and ..."

Dr. Pearson's list of questions goes on. And on. Didn't I answer all these on that new patient form in the waiting room already? Ugh! I answer as best I can, but I'm overwhelmed. He's asking about everything from how often I exercise to whether or not I eat breakfast. ***Does all this matter?*** Just tell me what's wrong with me!

The truth is, I'm scared–what if there ***is*** something seriously wrong, like a brain tumor!? Part of me wants to bring up my concern to the doctor; the other part doesn't even ***want*** to know, if that's the case. I fiddle nervously with the torn cuticle on my thumb. My hands are dry.

"Sorry, could you repeat that?" I say, suddenly realizing that Dr. Pearson has asked me a question and I've totally spaced.

***

"Of course," I say patiently. I can see that Michelle is getting overwhelmed by the questions. I also notice that she keeps squinting. "I asked how much caffeine you consume."

"I don't drink coffee."

"What about teas? Sodas?" I've had plenty of patients who down these drinks without realizing they contain caffeine.

"Oh yeah, I have a Coke sometimes." As she says the words, she squints up at the lights.

"Michelle, are you experiencing light sensitivity now?" I ask gently.

"Yes. That's usually the first sign a migraine is incoming."

"OK, let's dim these overheads." I lower my voice, realizing that she might also be more sensitive to noise. I usually speak up—a habit I have with my geriatric patients, who are often hard of hearing. But I keep my voice low as I continue asking Michelle questions.

Before digging into areas of improvement, it is important to highlight what is being done well in this exchange. There is some great evidence of solid EQ and accountability in action. Dr. Pearson's social awareness and responsiveness are illustrated when he picks up on Michelle's discomfort and adjusts the environment to accommodate her. They are further demonstrated in recognizing her concerns and providing reassurance that he is a peer and not looking to judge her. Michelle's self-awareness is highlighted by the fact that she recognizes her limitations from her evolving symptoms, but she continues to try to participate with honest responses. She realizes that even if she is nervous about details such as underage drinking, she has to be transparent with her GPS if she wants to get to her desired destination—a migraine-free life. However, when it comes to the history-taking element specifically, there are a few things that both sides could do better.

Information collected prior to the meeting doesn't seem to have been incorporated into Michelle's chart. Dr. Pearson then fires off a list of questions without framing their purpose or modifying their intensity after realizing Michelle appears unwell. Providing clarification on the relevance of certain questions can help a person feel more comfortable responding truthfully. On Michelle's side, she is trying her best, but she could advocate for herself by saying she isn't feeling well and that she's finding it hard to answer Dr. Pearson's questions as well as she would like. Unfortunately, these gaps risk the doctor having an incomplete picture of what is going on for her. A symptom diary used for one to two weeks prior to the appointment, tracking her migraines (when, where, how long) and accompanying symptoms, would be helpful, along with a record of her attempted treatments and lifestyle factors, such as diet, exercise, and sleep. This would provide a more reliable baseline from which to start formulating a care plan.

Finally, Michelle doesn't share her worries about a possible tumor with Dr. Pearson because she's afraid—if it *is* a tumor, she doesn't want to know. This kind of denial is not singular to Michelle's experience; I saw it in my mom's case. Pushing through such denial is an essential part of the history-taking process if patients are to reach their desired destination with their GPS.

History Is Always Subjective

For the HCP, history-taking is part of the clinical routine, yet it needs to be personalized to each encounter. When we ask certain questions, there is a method to our madness. Each question is used to inform the most likely diagnosis, giving direction as to what the HCP might expect to find in an examination and which tests or treatment, if any, are needed.

The history can be broad and comprehensive or brief and targeted, depending on the situation. It could include the following:

Chief complaint (CC)	**Reason why the person is presenting for care.**
History of presenting illness	Questions directed at creating a full picture of the details of the CC, or reason a person is seeking care.
Past medical history	Any previously diagnosed medical or psychiatric conditions. These can be either ongoing active conditions or resolved conditions.
Past surgical history	Any previous surgical procedures undergone.
Family medical history	Any known medical, psychiatric, neurological, or sleep disorders in a family member; the relationship to that family member; and, if known, age of onset, any related genetic testing, response to treatment, or related disability.
Social history	Home life and environment; relationship status and sexual habits; employment and/or school status; diet; alcohol; nicotine; or other substance use; reproductive history (may vary by age and location).
Medication history	Current medications, dosing, and indication; prior medications (as applicable).
Allergies	Any known food, medication, or environmental causes of physical reaction.
Review of systems	Questions directed at any other possible symptoms in different parts of the body that may help understand the lived experience and may have relevance or relation to the primary condition of concern.

To the patient, without context, some (if not many) of the topics covered may seem random or unnecessary. Among patients, there is a common yet erroneous belief that a diagnosis is only achieved through scans and tests. However, physicians are taught that the history makes the diagnosis; testing is used to support the diagnosis you already suspect based on the history. In most medical curricula, it is suggested that history accounts for 90 percent of the factors that will predict a likely diagnosis.

Much of my own experience of diagnosing and treating migraines comes through a pediatric lens. When concerned parents bring their child to a neurologist because of headaches, it is almost always with worry that the pain is due to something really bad, such as a brain tumor. This sets an expectation that imaging is necessary to exclude this concern. However, no one should be subjected to unnecessary diagnostic procedures that may lead to unnecessary anxiety, exposure to potential risk, or out-of-pocket expense.

The questions asked in such scenarios are guided by what possible causes may be responsible for the symptoms. Further questions are then refined by the responses given. All the while, the HCP is looking for red flags that could suggest that the child *does* need imaging—signs that this child is not experiencing a primary headache condition but something more worrisome, such as a tumor. More often than not, however, an MRI is not needed.

Communication Callout: Pediatric Medicine

History-taking takes on additional complexity for patients who are minors, whose parents or guardians are required to attend visits with them. When talking to older kids in particular—say tweens or teens—having Mom or Dad in the room for specific questions may not be ideal, especially if you have to ask about depression, suicidal thoughts, sex, drugs, alcohol, or even home life.

When these instances arise, I ask all the "parent-friendly" questions first, establishing communication and trust. I then state, "[Child's Name], as your doctor it is important to me to make sure you know I want to listen to you and understand what your thoughts are about what is going on. If it is OK, I would like to ask your parent/guardian to step out of the room temporarily. Is that OK?" If the patient agrees, I then ask the parent or guardian, "Would you mind if I spend a few minutes with [Child's Name] so that I can have an opportunity to speak with them alone and ensure I can listen to anything else they may want to share with me?" In most cases, both agree. If this is a telemedicine visit, I look to the patient to confirm that they are alone and can speak freely. There are other considerations to keep in mind with pediatric populations, of course—and we will look at those more closely in the next chapter, where our case study will feature a minor.

Sometimes, history-taking can be uncomfortable for the patient. Depending on the issue, HCPs may ask about everything from drugs to sex to bowel movements. Needless to say, sensitivity is a must.

Including explanations as to why such questions are relevant is helpful. Directness and honesty are always essential. This is why that meet-and-greet moment explored in the previous chapter is so critical—it lays the foundation of trust and respect upon which you can have a productive history-taking.

That said, history is *always* subjective. The HCP may have old patient records, which provide additional data. However, the primary source of information will be the history—and this will always be filtered through the lens of personal experience. HCPs must keep this in mind. To optimize history-taking, consider implementing these basic considerations:

- Provide context for the questions you are asking.
- Encourage honesty without judgment.
- Leave space for the patient to voice *their* concerns at any point by using open-ended questions such as, "Is there anything specific worrying you?"

If Dr. Pearson had asked Michelle this, she might have blurted out, "I'm afraid I have a brain tumor!" Figuring out what the patient's concern is allows you to collaboratively identify their unique treatment goals. It's the moment when they input their destination into the GPS so the GPS knows where to route them. I often use this GPS analogy with patients, and it has proven very useful in helping to create open communication.

Tools for History-Taking

A symptom diary is one of the most valuable history-taking tools any HCP and patient can use. I prefer to avoid disease-specific diaries, such as a "headache diary" or a "sleep diary," as these run the risk of excluding relevant symptoms because of their narrow focus. I therefore created a symptom diary that takes into consideration the entirety of a day, for a period of one or more weeks. It provides a longitudinal expression of what is being experienced, covering the timing, severity and frequency of symptoms, associated disability, sleep–wake scheduling, treatments tried, benefits experienced, and more.

Putting this into practice for someone with migraines could allow for a better understanding of symptom-specific points, such as when migraines occur, their severity and duration, associated disability, and the patient's response (did they eat, take medicine, nap?). It also makes space for recognized associated symptoms, such as nausea or vomiting. Further, it allows the patient to note any lifestyle factors that they may not associate with their migraine but which could be related, such as a stressful week of work or a sleepless night. Behavioral and lifestyle points to track could include school and work schedules, sleep schedules (including naps), meals (timing and content), and caffeine and alcohol intake. This information provides a great understanding of the individual's personalized baseline experience. A tailored therapeutic plan can then be implemented and monitored alongside the symptom diary—an approach to be discussed in future chapters.

Symptom Diary

SUNDAY	
Symptom(s)	Left-sided throbbing headache, difficulty concentrating, tired, feel dizzy/faint, restless broken sleep, nausea, sound-worsened headache
Onset and Offset	Terrible Night sleep—restless and woke up at 3am and had a hard time falling back to sleep, woke up feeling so tired and with mild headache; Headache—woke up with mild, left-side throbbing headache, skipped breakfast due to nausea; pain worsened at 1:30pm; Difficulty concentrating at work, took longer to complete work
Severity and Associate Disability	RBS—woke unrefreshed and maybe contributed to my headache; needed a nap; Headache—3/10—"can power through it" in AM, skipped breakfast b/c of HA and nausea; tried to avoid meds; worsened to 9/10 and conceded to take ibuprofen; difficulty concentrating—wanted to leave work, took longer to do work and quality not great, left work early to nap. Skipped dinner
Modifying Factors	Lots of coffee all day helped to feel more alert and also helped my headache some; Coffee made me feel less sleepy but worsened nausea and eventually headache; possibly new cleaning products at work made me feel like I was stabbed in eye; left work early to nap at 3:30pm, nap helped more than medication for my headache and was able to catch up on some work at home
Medication timing, dose and effects	ibuprofen 600mg 3pm when headache was 9/10, brought it down to 7/10

Sleep

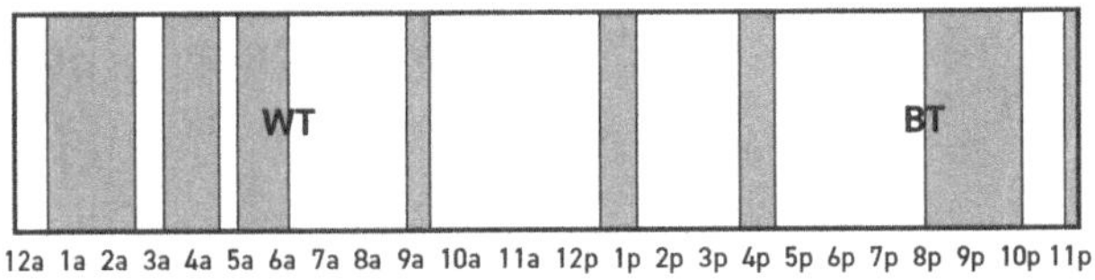

Figure 4.1: A sample symptom diary.

Symptom diaries provide infrastructure for accountability from both sides. For example, research has shown that a patient diary can be used to improve medicine adherence.[35] Another study suggests that, when used in outpatient care, symptom diaries help enhance patient engagement and reinforce the idea that patients are in control.[36] They also give the patient the ability to illustrate their experience to their HCP and determine together if it's a green light or if a detour is necessary.

Communication Callout: Support Persons

Social support is critical in any healthcare journey. Social support can come from family, significant others, friends, or other individuals with similar medical journeys. With this stated, it is not uncommon for a person to bring support with them to visits. Input from support systems can be critical to achieving the right diagnosis and treatment strategy. It requires balance to ensure that the patient is providing their history while also accepting input from their support person—without letting that support override or dismiss the patient's own contributions. As a person on a medical journey, have a discussion with your support system before your visit, articulating the role you would like them to play. How should (and shouldn't) they contribute? During the visit, let your HCP know what role you hope your support system can provide so they can share your expectation. As an HCP, always ask who is participating in the visit and clarify their role.

A symptom diary can also be helpful in establishing patterns of language used by the patient. Words matter! The lexicon of healthcare is likely very different from the words used in the broader community. When talking about something like migraine, for example, establishing clarity on the description of symptoms is necessary to ensure their accurate depiction. For an HCP, this may require asking the same question in different ways to ensure an accurate understanding. To understand the type of pain, the HCP might ask the following: "Describe the pain you experience. Is it stabbing? Is it tightness? Is it pulsating, like a heartbeat?" To determine the location of the pain, they might ask, "Where do you experience the pain?" as well as, "Can you point to where the pain typically occurs?" The symptom diary can help establish this level of detail.

There are also tech tools that can help with history-taking. In my medical institute, we're beginning to introduce ambient listening, an AI-powered scribe service. After a patient consents to the use of this software, their visit is conducted as usual—except, instead of being glued to the computer, feverishly typing notes, I am able to speak face-to-face with my patient without distraction. At the end of the visit, the software synthesizes an entire note based on the discussion, saving time and improving accuracy. In the future, I anticipate the ML algorithm will be able to recognize patterns in the symptoms as they are described and potentially suggest alternative or additional questions/considerations for diagnoses.

Finally, keep in mind that patient history is constantly developing. Both synchronous (at the time of the visit) and asynchronous (between-visit) history collection is necessary to achieve the right diagnosis and keep the course of care on the best track possible. This is why I emphasize that time is one of our best diagnostic tools. As an HCP, this feels incredibly uncomfortable because we are trained to believe that we are only as good as our ability to get the right answer on the first try. And for people experiencing a medical concern, this can augment feelings of vulnerability or doubt when an immediate diagnosis isn't provided. The truth is that there is more to gain through a continuous longitudinal care model where all relevant information is constantly shaping the patient's direction of care. Recording and assessing a person's habits and symptoms over weeks or months is sometimes necessary to achieve an accurate personalized diagnosis and therapeutic strategy.

A NARRATIVE CASE STUDY, REIMAGINED

Let's consider how Michelle's interaction with Dr. Pearson might have changed if both sides had implemented the best practices described in this chapter.

"So, Michelle, is there anything in particular that's concerning you today?"

"I'm worried about these migraines. I'm ... I'm scared it's a brain tumor." I expect Dr. Pearson to rush me off for a brain scan like in an episode of *Grey's Anatomy*. Instead, he says this:

"I appreciate your sharing your concern. That is very scary to think about. What I want you to hear me say is that migraines can have a *lot* of different contributors. Headaches related to a brain tumor typically have very specific characteristics as well as associated changes in the neurological exam that would prompt concern for the need for brain imaging. With all that said, let's discuss your experience more. Is there a history of brain tumors in your family?"

"I'm not sure." *Ugh.* I'm adopted. Do I need to share that with him? Is he going to ask questions?

"That's not a problem. Although a family history can be helpful, it is not uncommon that we may not have that information available to us. But this will not limit us from being able to better understand what you're experiencing. I would like to ask you some more questions."

I nod, relieved.

"Some of these questions might seem random to you, but they're all very useful in helping me to better understand your experience and inform the next steps we should take. Just answer as best you can and be honest. And it's OK if you aren't certain."

"OK."

He starts asking questions—just like he said, a lot of them seem random. He's asking about my sleep, eating, exercise, and more! Then he starts asking questions about the migraines.

"When was the last one? And do you know how long it lasted?"

This, at least, I'm ready for. I pull out my phone. "I actually have an app I use to track my migraines," I explain, feeling sort of silly.

"That's fantastic!" Dr. Pearson leans forward enthusiastically. "Could you give me the name? It may be useful for my other patients, too."

***

I make note of the app that Michelle mentions, happy to have found another tool that has helped Michelle feel empowered in her own journey—and that may help other patients. She fills me in on the details of her last few migraines using the app, which helps improve her accuracy in describing the events without biased recall.

With my AI transcription tool taking notes, I put my full focus on Michelle. I notice that she seems to squint at the overhead lights, so I ask if she is experiencing light sensitivity, which she confirms. I also notice that she keeps picking at her cuticles, which are dry and torn up—a sign of dehydration or anxiety? Both could certainly factor into her migraines. We should discuss behavioral and lifestyle factors and also introduce the idea of cognitive behavioral therapy.

By the time we've concluded our history-taking, Michelle and I have identified multiple lifestyle and behavioral factors that can be modified. We also discuss possible treatments for prevention and intervention for when Michelle has a headache. Together, we decide that, before starting any medication, it will be helpful for Michelle to keep a symptom and lifestyle diary for the next two weeks, especially with our new insights into possible contributing factors. I am also able to tell a relieved Michelle that her symptoms and neurological exam are reassuring and not indicative of a secondary cause of headache—meaning we don't need imaging right now. With a little more information and time, we'll be able to get Michelle to her migraine-free goal.

In this instance, Michelle and Dr. Pearson both come better prepared for the history-taking. Michelle has her app, while Dr. Pearson is more cognizant of setting the stage for the questions he's asking. He's also using a transcription tool so he can focus on Michelle. The end result—having Michelle implement a symptom diary—is a positive step in her healthcare journey. Although it can be tough when we don't figure it out right away, the truth is that personalized care requires time and continuous redirection.

COMMUNITY SUPPORT

Migraines can be extremely debilitating, making it difficult for people to perform everyday functions. The **American Migraine Foundation** and the **American Headache Society** are two excellent resources for patients, support networks, and HCPs alike. I've provided links to their pages in Appendix B.

With the patient's history complete, it's time to move on to the part of the process that some patients dislike—the exam. Every component of the interaction prior to this has been helping to build up to a successful exam: from establishing trust in the meet-and-greet to encouraging transparency during history-taking. Still, the exam can be stressful for many and has unique considerations of its own.

Growth Opportunity: Time for a History Lesson

As with the meet-and-greet, when it comes to history-taking, there are things both the HCP and the patient can do to improve the process. For HCPs, I recommend opening history-taking with one simple question: "What concerns brought you here today?" Create space for the patient to voice this so you can help them articulate the destination for their GPS. For patients, I recommend a symptom diary; the QR code below links to a template symptom diary you can use.

Chapter 4 Endnotes

35 M. van Berge Henegouwen, H. van Driel, and D. Kasteleijn-nolst trenité, "A Patient Diary as a Tool to Improve Medicine Compliance," *Pharmacy World and Science* 21 (1999): 21–24, https://doi.org/10.1023/A:1008627824731.

36 Bryan Hodge, "The Use of Symptom Diaries in Outpatient Care," *Family Practice* 20, no. 3 (2013): 24–28, https://www.aafp.org/pubs/fpm/issues/2013/0500/p24.html.

CHAPTER 5

Exam Time

The purpose of this chapter is to consider an interaction where proactive communication may not be considered—the exam. For the HCP, this is business as usual. However, physical maneuvers and evaluations without explanation, or even an unanticipated "hmmm" or surprised look during an assessment, can be a source of anxiety, dread, and even embarrassment for a patient. Expectation-setting regarding what may be done, an explanation of its relevance, and even a summary of both the reassuring or potentially concerning findings help build a trusting relationship.

NARRATIVE CASE STUDY: A CONCERNED PARENT TAKES THEIR DAUGHTER FOR A CHECKUP

Sarah is a nineteen-year-old woman with autism spectrum disorder and intellectual disability, and she is nonverbal. Her mother, Jennifer Goldman, is her primary caregiver and legal guardian. Jennifer has brought Sarah to Dr. Bolton for a checkup.

Dr. Bolton is a primary care physician who is new to Sarah, and he is establishing care now that Sarah has "graduated" from her pediatrician. As the exam approaches, Jennifer becomes anxious.

I try to keep calm. I've already reviewed my daughter's medical history with Dr. Bolton. But now it's time for the actual exam. And anxious thoughts are racing through my mind: *The last time I brought Sarah to a new provider, it didn't go well. Sarah's sensitivity to others touching her posed a major challenge for Dr. Frost. He ended up agitated, and Sarah became overwhelmed. She started to become aggressive, requiring me to physically get in between them and ask to stop the exam before we risked her becoming combative. It took days for her to settle after that. I hope today goes better.*

Dr. Bolton has already greeted us both. I'm grateful that he acknowledged not only me but also Sarah. Not everyone does. With the formalities done, it's time to get started.

"Mrs. Goldman, thank you for bringing Sarah in today. I appreciate your being here for the exam. Is it OK for you if we get started?"

"Yes, thank you." I nod.

Dr. Bolton directs his attention to Sarah. "Sarah, I need to examine you now to make sure you're healthy. Is that OK?"

I watch as Sarah fidgets in her seat.

"To do the exam, I need you to get on the table, Sarah."

Sarah looks intently away.

Dr. Bolton repeats the request for Sarah to get on the table and then glares at me, as if expecting me to move her onto the table. Fears of

Sarah becoming agitated flood my head, and sweat begins to collect on my brow. Thankfully, Sarah then jumps on the table.

"I'd like to start by listening to Sarah's lungs with the stethoscope." Dr. Bolton holds up his shiny stethoscope. "Sarah, this is a stethoscope. It's something I use to listen to your lungs to make sure they're healthy. To do that, I have to hold it to your chest and your back, here and here." He points on his own body. "The stethoscope might feel cold, but it doesn't hurt, OK?"

Sarah watches Dr. Bolton but doesn't acknowledge what he's said.

"Maybe you'd like to touch the stethoscope first to see what it feels like," Dr. Bolton goes on.

"That's probably a good idea," I say quickly. "Sarah hates the cold."

"That makes two of us, Sarah," Dr. Bolton says with a smile. "I love the summer, but I don't like winter. But the stethoscope isn't that cold, see?" Dr. Bolton holds out the stethoscope and touches his finger to the metal. "You can touch it, if you want."

Sarah diverts her gaze again.

"Maybe Mom wants to touch it first to test it out," the doctor suggests.

I reach out and touch the cool metal, which Dr. Bolton has already warmed up slightly in his hand. "Oh, that's not so bad. Sarah, do you want to touch it?" As I ask her, I kneel down to meet her gaze–she's still looking at the floor. Hesitantly, she reaches out and touches the stethoscope.

This is already going better than the last appointment we had, which felt rushed. I give Dr. Bolton a relieved smile. ***Maybe this won't be so bad!***

***

The introduction with Sarah and her mom goes well enough. But now I'm trying to get Sarah to breathe deeply for me, inhale and exhale, and she isn't cooperating.

"Just in and out, Sarah," I say for what feels like the twentieth time. I stand in front of her and demonstrate, inhaling and exhaling slowly. She just looks the other way. But she's also getting more fidgety. I'm worried if we don't get this done soon, we won't get it done at all.

"OK, let's try again." I place the stethoscope on Sarah's chest. Up until now, she's been fine with the touch. But this time, she swats my hand away.

"Sarah!" Mrs. Goldman admonishes her with a shocked tone. "I'm sorry," she adds, turning to me.

"Not a problem," I say, forcing a smile. "I tell you what. How about we move ahead with some other parts of the exam, and we can try this again at the end."

I don't want to put pressure on Sarah and cause her to be more uncomfortable than she already is. But I'm also losing hope that I'll be able to complete this exam—and I am hesitant to try other parts of the exam, as I don't want her to become combative. I was planning to have her seen by gynecology because her mom described some irregular bleeding over the past six months. But if I can't even listen to Sarah's lungs, a gynecological exam is certainly not going to be possible. We will put that on the back burner and continue to monitor her symptoms for now.

This is going to be a tough one ...

Individualizing our approaches to exams is critical. We're typically taught that our approach to an exam should be guided by the chief complaint and the patient history. This may result in either a very focused examination of a single or a select number of organ systems, or a more detailed and comprehensive exam. Over my career, I have learned that the exam needs to be adapted based not only on the history but also on the age and specific needs of the individual and their comfort levels.

Individuals with neurodivergence may have unique needs that require an adjustment, such as stereotyped self-stimulatory behaviors, sensory processing challenges, impulse control challenges, and even aggressive behavior. Pediatric training provides exposure to a range of individual needs and relevant techniques. Because of the constant exposure to different developmental stages, pediatric clinicians typically require patience, distraction techniques, and even a softness to their interactions that makes them feel approachable.

Dr. Bolton does quite a few things very well in this interaction. First, although Dr. Bolton has never met Sarah, he enters the examination attempting to engage both Sarah and her mother. Just because a patient is nonverbal does not mean they are not to be addressed. Dr. Bolton exemplifies this, addressing not only Sarah's mother but also Sarah. It's communication 101, but when someone is nonverbal or unable to respond, this basic step sometimes gets lost. Even when a patient is in a coma, I introduce myself, put my hand on their shoulder or forehead, and say that I am sorry they are so ill; I also let them know what I'm doing as I'm doing it.

Second, Dr. Bolton doesn't rush Sarah. He looks for physical cues of anxiety and is careful to pause and step back when he senses frustration. This is an opportunity to re-engage Sarah's mother for assistance or recommendations on what may have been helpful in the past. He suggests they revisit the part of the exam that Sarah is visibly disinterested in and even agitated by at the end. Medical education typically places a strong emphasis on a structured approach to examinations, with each step taken in a given order. Sometimes, it's necessary to step outside of this scheme.

Still, Sarah's participation comes to a halt. A physical exam often requires a patient to follow instructions, from touching their toes to breathing deeply. In Sarah's case, Dr. Bolton struggles to guide her through the deep breathing needed to check her lungs. Unfortunately, the impact of this not only discourages the anticipation of success for the remainder of the exam but also spills over to affect other planned care needs—the gynecological exam. This is an important illustration of the domino effect of failed communication.

This is an instance in which the parent's or companion's assistance could be useful. Even when a person is without cognitive or verbal disability, there are times when a family member or companion can advocate for options in the examination that may make it more tolerable for the patient. When we revisit the narrative case study at this chapter's conclusion, we'll look again at how a support person's participation can make a difference.

The Basis for a Successful Exam

My journey in healthcare has been and continues to be guided by five foundational principles: **trust**, **respect**, **communication**, **best-in-class care**, and **teamwork**. The need for each of these components is exemplified by the patient–HCP interaction during the exam.

Take something as personal as a genitalia exam during a gynecologic appointment or a rectal exam with a specialist. The intrusive nature of these examinations can create tension and even avoidance behaviors, resulting in enhanced health risk due to lack of care. Unfortunately, this is too frequently observed in adults with intellectual disability. This underscores the foundational importance of trust and respect from the meet-and-greet and the need for ongoing and transparent communication to bolster trust, respect, and willing partnership. This, in combination with attention to individual needs, results in best-in-class personalized care. HCPs should specify at every step what they are doing and why. If for any reason there is a gap, the patient or their support system should query it, expressing whether the patient is interested, concerned, or fearful. Shared responsibility from all sides is needed.

Set the stage for success with the five *W*'s:

- **Who:** Who is doing the exam? Will another person be in the room? A doctor may ask to have a third party (chaperone) in the room for safety and comfort during sensitive parts of the exam, such as a breast or genital examination. Patients can also request to have a chaperone—or, alternatively, to have learners excused from the room for privacy.
- **What:** What are the medical and nonmedical terms used to describe the exam or the findings? What are you looking for, and how will this inform what may be occurring? What is considered normal or abnormal? What is expected of the patient? Is there a need for disrobing or wearing a gown? What should be expected at each step of the exam? For example, if the doctor is going to listen to the patient's heart and wants to have the stethoscope against the skin and not the shirt, they may explain why and ask permission.

- **When:** Depending on circumstance, the timing of the examination may occur out of sequence from what is typically performed. For instance, if the patient is a baby who is due to eat, an examination may be done before the history is complete to avoid excessive movements right after eating. Setting expectations for how long the exam may take is also helpful and can ease tension or awareness, especially during any sensitive parts.
- **Where:** Can the exam be done in the current setting? Will there be more than one setting for evaluation? Does the patient need to stand, sit, or lie down? Will there be any special equipment used for the examination? For instance, during an ophthalmology appointment, there may be more than one room that the patient is examined in, and some parts of the exam may be performed by the clinician's team members. Introduction of the team member, their credentials, and what they are doing keeps the patient informed.
- **Why:** Why are you performing the exam? Or, equally important, why are you not performing parts of the exam? The level of detail discussed may vary on a case-by-case basis.

The communication does not stop after the exam, of course. Typically, a summary of the history and physical exam findings, both reassuring and concerning features, serves as a great foundation to begin a discussion of the assessment and plan.

Communication Callout: Learners in the Room

In many clinical settings, learners may be present. These can include new hires, trainees, or even volunteers who aspire to go into medicine. This represents an important educational opportunity for teaching both examination skills and communication strategies. Typically, I will ask the patient and family if it is OK to discuss the examination and findings out loud to teach the learners. I will explain that I will use medical terms to describe what I am doing or what I find but that I will also discuss this in nonmedical terms so that all of us understand what I am saying. I might conclude with something like, "At any time, if you have any questions or are uncomfortable, please let me know. It is important that we all stay on the same page." In these situations, it is important to monitor the patient's comfort, especially if the learner is performing the exam. As a patient, it's always possible to ask that learners not be involved, either at all or in specific capacities.

In cases involving minors or adults with impaired cognitive function or other specific anticipatory needs, the communication needs become even greater. Does a parent or guardian need to be in the room? Should a third-party chaperone be present? Are there other limitations that are not known or visible to the examiner? How is the process being communicated—and contextualized, considering the patient's life in general? For a child, a doctor might reiterate the ideas of safe touch and physical boundaries by explaining, "I'm going to look at your private area. This is something that, as a doctor, I am doing because I am making sure you are healthy. However, other people should not look at or touch these areas. It is important if you are ever uncertain that you tell your parents or an adult you trust." These discussions are also an opportunity to observe for any cues that may imply abuse or neglect.

The goal is always best-in-class care. However, detours may prevent or delay this—as we see in Dr. Bolton's decision to push back Sarah's gynecological exam. In such instances, it's important to remember that every patient has a history other than their medical history. There is also an emotional and mental history, held internally, that the HCP may not be privy to. As such, there may be a preconditioned response to what is happening that you are unaware of—but that you can better prepare yourself to empathetically respond to. This is an exercise of your social awareness and your social management abilities: to redirect the course even when an unexpected detour occurs, further personalizing the journey at every turn.

Communication Callout: Bias

There are numerous biases that can occur in medicine and interfere with the ability to achieve best-in-class care. For instance, in a high-volume ER where there has been a historical issue of drug-seeking behavior and concerns about the risks associated with opioid prescribing, there may be a heightened degree of skepticism regarding who would "qualify" to receive more than non-steroidal anti-inflammatory medications. If a patient presents with pain in the ER and is seeking medication, will their pain be optimally treated? Or will that patient perhaps be perceived as drug-seeking? Research has demonstrated that when patients request opioid pain medications, physicians are more likely to suspect they are drug-seeking.[37] This may result

> in undertreating pain, possibly forcing that patient to go to another ER—which skews the optics further.
>
> Despite ongoing concerns regarding opioids, optimal management of the patient's concerns is still a necessity. Awareness of these biases shouldn't lead a physician to go against their instinct to avoid opioids, but instead introduces an opportunity for them to create a new path for pain management. In fact, strategic opioid use and preferentially non-opioid medication-based pathways have been successfully illustrated and modeled in pre-hospital care and emergency rooms internationally.[38] Bias awareness introduces the opportunity to turn potential crises into creativity, allowing the patient to more successfully continue to move forward on their journey.

The problem is that medicine is still rarely taught from a person-first approach. Although an increasing number of schools have introduced case-based learning, the focus for the first two years of school is still largely on gaining scientific knowledge, typically taught through classroom didactics. In the last two years of medical school, there are clinical rotations that allow for a medical student to interact with people who are on their medical journeys. However, the focus is less on how the student interacts and more so on how they report the information collected. The only time interaction tends to be called out is when it is heinously apparent that professionalism is lacking.

As a doctor of osteopathic medicine (a DO), a person-first approach was a critical aspect of my education. In fact, a scolding would be the response to a student who led with disease-first language such as "the hypertensive patient" or "the epileptic." Instead, I was taught to lead with the person experiencing the disorder, so "Mr.

Johnson with refractory hypertension" or "Jennie, a spunky five-year-old girl, with well-controlled absence seizures." Too often, HCPs fixate on medicine first, at the expense of the human component. This contributes to a disconnect in communication and can significantly impact efforts in care, including the exam.

From the patient's side, the exam is typically expected when receiving care, but there is generally no understanding of how it contributes to medical decision-making. This can result in an unanticipated disconnect, as each clinical situation may demand different exam approaches. As a society, we have been conditioned since early childhood to expect that good care equals, at minimum, a stethoscope on the chest; if this doesn't occur, especially without explanation, it may lead to doubt and distrust.

For example, I have received a parental complaint about a member of my team's evaluation of their child, who was experiencing headaches. The parent stated that they did not trust my team member's assessment of migraine as the diagnosis and still wanted an MRI of the brain for their child. They felt my team member had cut corners and missed something that would warrant an MRI. In fact, as I reviewed the child's history and examination, I reaffirmed my team member's findings. The patient was a teenager whose headaches had classic features of migraine with aura and had recently increased in frequency and severity in the context of restrictive eating for weight loss, an erratic sleep schedule due to many school and extracurricular commitments, and a related increase in caffeine use. The neurological exam was detailed, highlighting pertinent negative findings that provided significant reassurance against any type of secondary pathology, such as a brain tumor. An MRI was not warranted.

In this particular situation, it was my job to bridge the communication gap. I did not belittle or discount my team member's decision-making, nor did I dismiss or minimize the parent's concerns. I first acknowledged the issue and apologized, then communicated my own concerns, and finally empathized with how devastating it must feel, as a parent, to witness their child suffering and worry that something has been missed. The parent's response: a sigh in agreement. After establishing a foundation built on a mutual understanding of their concern, I re-examined the information with the parents, summarized the findings, and explained the rationale around the decision-making. We agreed upon steps for managing the headaches, defined the metrics of success to use, and pinpointed signs or symptoms that would redirect us to needing imaging. I closed the discussion with the most important statement: "You now have a whole team to partner with that also wants the best for your child. We are here to support you both while we work toward optimal headache control."

In the end, this all comes back to that big piece of the puzzle we talked about in the earlier chapters: EQ. Awareness of self and others, and how we manage what we are perceiving. Are the actions the HCP performs in an exam being perceived by the patient as they are intended? Are the words coming across as desired? Is the message landing?

The same question can be asked of the patient. Again, this is a two-way street, with accountability needed on both sides. If the patient has concerns about the exam, are they giving voice to these? If they are uncomfortable with part of the exam, are they speaking up? If they want a third party in the room, be that a nurse or a language interpreter or a friend or family member, are they expressing this need?

HCPs can't be mind-readers, but they can pick up on physical cues of discomfort. For example, when palpating a patient's abdomen, they may notice the patient wince or cringe in pain. However, what if the patient is a stoic who doesn't want to shy away? Words are needed. Both sides must communicate. It's a team effort. That's why teamwork is the final word in my personal guiding mantra, as both a physician and a human being.

Support for a Successful Exam

One reason why teamwork is so important in the exam is that both the HCP and the patient are up against some unfortunate and unavoidable systemic issues—time being one of the biggest. On one hand, clinicians must balance the consistent pressure to see people quickly with seeing them appropriately in order to provide the best care. On the other hand, there may be instances when an exam needs to be abbreviated to facilitate an expedited path forward. For instance, say I'm consulting with a patient and note signs of a neurological condition that warrants immediate action. Completing the remainder of the exam before addressing a potentially life-altering concern could be a risky move. In these situations, a calm discussion briefly summarizing my concerns and laying out next steps is necessary to keep the patient informed and reassured. And then we move on to whatever those next steps may be, communicating all the while. Personalized care is putting the person as the focus of every step of the interaction.

The standard approach to examination is taught in medical school; it is usually structured by the organ system from head to toe. However, it is infrequently taught that we should explain to the person being examined what we are doing, why we are doing it, and how what we are doing is influencing our assessment as we go through it. There is nothing wrong, in principle, with taking a systemic approach to an exam—something like a checklist is useful, keeping the exam on track and ensuring no details are missed. However, being capable of confidently stepping *outside* the checklist to personalize evaluations when needed is critical. Say a patient tells you that they develop certain symptoms when they go running. You probably wouldn't find this in your checklist, but you could ask them to run up and down the exam room to try to elicit those symptoms. A patient might say, "Are you crazy?! You want me to run around in here?" Explain that you are attempting to recreate the patient's symptoms to reveal a finding during the examination that isn't present when evaluating the patient at rest—and that this may give better insight into the cause of the concern and reduce the number of unnecessary tests or referrals.

Adapting exams could also mean adjusting the sequence of steps in your checklist or adjusting how you perform the actual procedure. Although this book's chapters are ordered according to the typically expected sequence of interactions, it has been purposely designed so that each chapter can also be read independently. HCPs and patients can likewise go "out of order." As an HCP, if you need to start the examination before a detailed history—for example, because of urgency—you should. As a patient or support person, if you want to get a certain part of the exam done sooner rather than later, say so. Being able to adapt the exam or asking for adaptations when you have specific needs are both equally necessary.

Communication Callout: Pediatric Patients

Flexibility can be especially relevant for a pediatric patient or a special-needs patient like Sarah. If I enter the exam room and I see a child is fighting sleep, and Mom tells me, "It's almost nap time," I do the exam first. This way, if the child falls asleep, I don't have to wake them—I can still take their history by talking to the parent. And the way the exam looks may be different, too. With a young child, an exam may consist of playtime—skipping and jumping with the other person, playing peekaboo, you name it. While I'm "playing," I'm really observing. And the parent can play a big part in inciting action and playing along, freeing up my attention so it can remain on the patient. I will also verbalize summaries of what I am observing and will confirm if what I am seeing is consistent with what is seen at home or if it's a feature of concern. It is critical that my patients and their families verify my findings. Otherwise, I run the risk of an erroneous assessment and a mismatch of expectations of care. It takes teamwork.

A successful exam requires communication at every stage, from preparation to follow-up. These exam checklists for HCPs and patients cover some communication essentials.

EXAM COMMUNICATION CHECKLIST FOR HCPS

Before the exam:

- Have you checked whether the patient has any special needs, such as a need for an interpreter, or preferences, such as having a third party in the room?

- Have you conveyed the five *W*'s of your exam? Who is doing it? What is being done? When is it being done? Where is it being done? Why and how is it being done?
- Have you asked the patient if they have any questions or concerns?
- Have you prepared your team? If a third party is going to be in the room, what is their role? What should they be doing before, during, and after the exam?

During the exam:

- Have you reiterated the five *W*'s?
- Have you adapted the exam as needed–including to elicit the necessary symptoms? For instance, if the patient's symptoms appear only after they climb stairs ... find some stairs!
- Are you narrating the exam as you go, confirming or negating what you're seeing (e.g., based on the history)?
- Are you checking in with your patient physically, looking for signs of discomfort or pain?
- Are you checking in with your patient verbally? ("Any discomfort?" "Any pain?" "Does it hurt when I press here?")
- Are you paying attention? Often, I see people doing exams and just going through the mechanical motions, not noticing cues such as the patient wincing in pain.
- Are you seeking feedback as you go through the exam? Your patient is the expert in their body. They know what is and isn't normal for them.

After the exam:

- What's next? Communicate future steps.

I have included a QR code to a printable version of this checklist at the chapter's conclusion.

Here's the patient version.

EXAM COMMUNICATION CHECKLIST FOR PATIENTS

Before the exam:

- Do you have any special needs your HCP may not know about, e.g., do you want a third party in the room, or do you want to bring a friend or family member? Do you require an interpreter? Do you require any sort of assistive technology?
- Do you know the five *W*'s of your exam? Who is doing it? What is being done? When is it being done? Where is it being done? Why and how is it being done?
- Are there any questions or concerns about the exam you haven't yet expressed?
- Are you comfortable? Is there anything the HCP can do to make you more comfortable, such as washing their hands again?

During the exam:

- Are any questions coming up for you during the exam? Are you asking them?
- Are any symptoms arising during the exam? Are you communicating these to your doctor?
- Are you in physical or mental pain or discomfort at any point? Have you expressed this verbally?
- Is there a part of the exam you are not comfortable doing, physically or mentally?
- "Press pause" when needed.

After the exam:

- What's next? Clarify future steps.

In the case of virtual exams, these checklists may need to be adapted. Telemedicine is becoming increasingly normalized, which has distinct benefits for patient access. There is a growing number of digital technologies and innovations that are allowing for more at-home diagnostics and care than in the past. This creates the ongoing need for adaptability—from HCPs, patients, and health systems alike—as approaches to exam and overall healthcare delivery evolve.

For instance, currently, if my child is complaining of ear pain, tugging at their ear and appearing ill, I will take him to the pediatrician for evaluation of an ear infection. A pediatrician will use a specialized piece of equipment called an otoscope to look in the ear and see if there are signs of infection, such as fluid behind the tympanic membrane, or ear drum. An even more confirmatory effort would include insufflation—while looking at the ear, small puffs of air are applied to see if the eardrum moves. Now, what would be great was if these ear infections always started between nine in the morning and five in the evening Monday to Friday! However, these symptoms seem to always happen at two o'clock on a Saturday morning.

Enter a digital application that is directed at solving this problem: WavelyDx. This is a cell phone–based application that can diagnose ear infections. A small paper cone is attached to a cell phone and then placed in the patient's ear canal. It creates a sound in the ear and, within seconds, based on the acoustic feedback, responds with a high or low likelihood of infection. This approach carries a sensitivity and specificity that closely resembles the performance of a pediatrician. In other words, the research shows that this is an accurate and reliable method, which is why it's received FDA clearance. This enables my family to confidently be screened, even at two o'clock on a Saturday morning. If the result is positive, we can set up a telemedicine appointment or even send in a summary of symptoms and a screenshot of the test results to help expedite care. In addition to convenience, it may also help reduce unnecessary antibiotics and minimize variability in the care delivered.

There's a lot of promise in these kinds of advancements. However, it's also important to know when remote is not enough. Telemedicine can be a good first step in connecting with the patient, offering a lower barrier to entry. But some types of exams—and subsequent assessments and tests—may need to be done face-to-face.

Whether it's in person or via a video call, communication is a must both before and during exam time. Adequate preparation and expectation-setting for a successful examination will lead to more optimal interactions and exam success. Particular attention to individualizing this based on different communication needs is essential. A patient with special needs, such as Sarah, is going to have a different experience. Adaptability is essential.

A NARRATIVE CASE STUDY, REIMAGINED

When we left Dr. Bolton and Sarah in the exam room at the start of the chapter, Dr. Bolton was struggling to get Sarah to inhale and exhale so he could listen to her lungs. Let's see how things might look different with support from Sarah's mom.

Sarah isn't breathing like Dr. Bolton has requested, and I can see that the doctor is getting frustrated. I wring my hands anxiously—and then I have an idea.

"Dr. Bolton, maybe I can try something?" I ask tentatively. I don't want him to think I'm overstepping.

"Of course! Please. You know Sarah best. I welcome your help!" He steps back.

I address my daughter. "Sarah, remember how we celebrated your birthday last week? And you got the chocolate cake with all the candles?"

Sarah keeps fidgeting, but I can tell that she's paying attention to me. Her movements slow slightly.

"You blew out the candles, right? And you took a big breath in and out to do it?" I mimic the action. "Can you show Dr. Bolton how you did it?"

***

Thank God for moms like this one. I smile as Sarah joins her mom in blowing out her imaginary birthday candles. This is a trick for me to remember for next time, and it may help some of my other patients, too.

"That's great, Sarah! Can you show me again?" As Sarah continues, I am able to listen to her lungs with my stethoscope, getting nice deep inhales and exhales for a more comprehensive and accurate assessment.

When we're done, I turn to Mrs. Goldman. "Thank you! That was very helpful. In the future, please know that I always welcome your guidance. You and Sarah are the experts in what helps her to best participate and feel comfortable. Together, we will make a great team to keep her healthy."

I can see the relief on Mrs. Goldman's face.

"There are a few other parts of the exam that might be challenging. Maybe you can help me with those as well," I suggest, thinking of the gynecologic exam I was hoping to refer Sarah for. Mrs. Goldman nods. This is going to be a team effort.

Here, rather than getting frustrated and skipping this part of the exam, Dr. Bolton takes a different tactic: Ask Mom! Mrs. Goldman knows Sarah better than Dr. Bolton ever can. She lives with Sarah and has cared for her since birth. In this case, we see how that connection can be leveraged to help the exam go more smoothly. By referring to the birthday candles, Mom is able to guide Sarah appropriately, supporting Dr. Bolton in the exam while maintaining Sarah's comfort.

Play to the strategy the patient knows. This applies in any exam context, for any patient. As we saw with a pediatric patient, having Mom or Dad help demonstrate a task—whether it's breathing in and out, skipping, or hopping on one leg—can provide successful guidance. The parent has a background with the child; the child trusts them. Make the most of that strength. Tap into the power of the team.

COMMUNITY SUPPORT

The need for community—a team—is critically important for those with autism or neurodevelopmental divergence (NDD). There are a number of advocacy organizations that support individuals with autism and NDD and their caregivers. I suggest looking to **Autism Speaks**, the **Autism Society**, the **Simons Foundation Autism Research Initiative**, and the **Colin Farrell Foundation**. You will find links to each of these in Appendix B.

Everything we've covered up until now, from the exam to the history-taking, is leading to the next chapter: assessment and options. This can be an emotionally charged moment, even when communication has been thorough and collaborative thus far. How can HCPs and patients alike prepare for a potential mismatch of expectations? And what happens if the HCP's final assessment is "I don't know?"

> **Growth Opportunity: Your Exam Communication Checklist**
>
> Both the patient and the HCP have to participate in the exam. What can you do in ***your*** role to make sure it's a success? I've included links to the communication checklists from this chapter below. These are printable versions you can use and share—for example, HCPs may want to give these to their patients.

Chapter 5 Endnotes

37 Michael A. Fischer, John B. McKinlay, Jeffrey N. Katz, Eric Gerstenberger, Felicia Trachtenberg, Lisa D. Marceau et al., "Physician Assessments of Drug Seeking Behavior: A Mixed Methods Study," *PLoS One* 12, no. 6 (2023): e0178690, https://doi.org/10.1371/journal.pone.0178690.

38 George Lindbeck, Manish I. Shah, Sabina Braithwaite, Jonathan R. Powell, Ashish R. Panchal, Lorin R. Brown et al., "Evidence-Based Guidelines for Prehospital Pain Management: Recommendations," *Prehospital Emergency Care* 27, no. 2 (2025): 144–153, https//doi.org/10.

1080/10903127.2021.2018073; Saïd Hachimi-Idrissi, Viliam Dobias, Wolf E. Hautz, Robert Leach, Thomas C. Sauter, Idanna Sforzi et al., "Approaching Acute Pain in Emergency Settings; European Society for Emergency Medicine (EUSEM) Guidelines—Part 2: Management and Recommendations," *Internal Emergency Medicine* 15, no. 7 (2020): 1141–1155, https://doi.org/10.1007/s11739-020-02411-2.

CHAPTER 6

Assessment and Available Options

The purpose of this chapter is to remind both the HCP and the patient to circle back to the initial goals of their interaction. Take a beat to reflect. Were the objectives met? For the patient, their goals are what they input into their GPS for their healthcare journey; the GPS is supposed to help them get there. For that to happen, it's essential to revisit those goals and consider next steps, in line with the assessment and available options.

NARRATIVE CASE STUDY: A PERSON WITH ASTHMA IN THE ER, AGAIN

Jonas is living with asthma. He was diagnosed six months ago and immediately put on medication by Dr. Nelson because of the severity of his asthma. Although Jonas is taking his medication, he keeps ending up in the ER. What Jonas doesn't realize is that his "stretching" of his meds to make them last for more than a month, due to cost concerns, is making the meds less effective—and is putting him at risk.

I can't believe I'm back here. It's my third time in the ER this month. But Dr. Nelson said that I should always come to the ER if I feel like I can't breathe. I just did what he said. Here he is now.

"Hi Jonas, I see you had an asthma attack. How are you feeling now?"

"Better. I mean, I can breathe again." I'm still exhausted.

"Good, I'm glad to hear that. But I am concerned that this is your third time in the ER this month. That can't be fun."

"Nah, and I'm missing work, too." I don't mention that I've missed so much work I'm in danger of getting fired—which would be bad, because then I'd lose the insurance that pays for my meds. Well, it kind of pays for them. The co-pay is really high. But I usually manage to stretch out the use to about six weeks by doing one puff of my inhaler instead of two most mornings. "But I knew I had to come in. I needed my emergency inhaler like every hour! And you said that I should come in if I need it more than every two hours."

"You were absolutely right to come in. Like I said, if you need the blue inhaler more than every two hours, head straight to the ER. That said, we don't want your asthma interfering with your daily life." Dr. Nelson shakes his head. "I want to make sure we've got your meds right. Do you have them and your spacer with you?"

"Yup." I reach for my bag where I keep the inhalers and the spacer. "I brought them with me to the ER, like you said I should if this happens."

"Good, good." Dr. Nelson looks pleased. "So, you've got the blue inhaler and the red one. When are you taking which one? And how often?"

"I take the red one every morning, like you said, and before bed at night. And the blue one is for emergencies only." Does he think I'm dumb or something?

"That's good. Can you maybe show me how you use them—try the blue one."

I demonstrate as Dr. Nelson watches. I feel sort of like an animal at the zoo. Why is he making me do all this?

***

I watch as Jonas administers his inhaler. Sometimes, patients struggle with this, in which case I'll have an asthma nurse come demonstrate for him. But he's doing everything right. "How many puffs do you normally take?" I ask when he's done.

"Two." Jonas eyes me suspiciously. Suddenly, I realize I've been asking him to jump through hoops without explaining why. Rookie mistake.

"That's the perfect amount. Jonas, the reason I'm asking these questions is that I want to make sure I've prescribed the right medications for you. Sometimes, the medications are the right ones, but patients can have trouble taking them the right way. I just want to rule that possibility out so we can make sure you don't end up in the ER again."

"Got it, Doc." Jonas seems to relax. After a pause, he adds, "It would be good to figure this out. I keep missing work, and I need that for my insurance so ... Yeah." He trails off awkwardly.

"I hear you, Jonas. I want to figure this out too." I keep my tone optimistic but, honestly, I'm confused. From what I can tell, Jonas is doing everything right. He's taking the medication with a spacer to improve delivery at the right time, in the right amount. He's even a model patient, remembering to bring his meds and spacer with him when he comes into the ER.

> But he's still ending up here every other week. I'm going to have to escalate his preventative inhaler–maybe that will better control his symptoms and keep him out of the ER.

In Jonas's scenario, we are seeing a patient who has been successfully diagnosed and has his treatment seemingly at his fingertips. As a person living with asthma, Jonas has a reactive airway that responds inappropriately to certain stimuli—the bronchioles basically clamp down, making it harder for air to move through the lungs and for oxygen to get into the blood. To manage his asthma, Jonas has both a controller and a rescue medication.

Controller medications are used to prevent an exacerbation of a disorder—in this case, an asthma exacerbation or attack. Rescue medications are used as needed when there are symptoms or episodic worsening of a condition. The frequency of use of the rescue medication dictates whether or not the controller medication is appropriate. If a patient requires their rescue medication multiple times a week or day, this can indicate a need to start or escalate a controller medication.

One of the biggest challenges with some of these medications is how their use is coordinated. First, there's the question of differentiating between the controller and the rescue medication; this can be confusing, especially to new patients, as they can look almost identical. Then, there is the fact that the patient needs to coordinate breathing in and pumping the asthma inhaler at the same time—otherwise, the medication lands on their tongue and doesn't go into the lungs, where it's needed. Frequently, an aerochamber or spacer can be used to improve delivery of this medication, boosting its efficacy.

Dr. Nelson and Jonas are both doing a lot of things well in this exchange. Jonas took note of the danger sign that Dr. Nelson flagged—needing his emergency inhaler more than every two hours. When that sign popped up, he went to the ER and brought his meds and spacer with him. Meanwhile, Dr. Nelson is confirming that Jonas has the right meds and is taking them the right way, at the right time. He even considers whether an asthma nurse might be needed to demonstrate proper medication usage but decides it's not necessary.

However, Jonas may end up with an unnecessary escalation of therapy because of a lack of discussion about stretching out the use of his medication because of cost. Access to medications that are cost-prohibitive for optimal adherence is common and frequently unrecognized if it is not discussed. If the co-pay is too high, not getting the medication at all or "stretching" medications when feeling less ill to make them last longer is a possibility. The result? Inadequate dosing—leading to lack of improvement and even increased exacerbations, like Jonas's.

Assessing for the Patient, Not for the Disease

The need to look at the whole patient applies across the board, not just for those with asthma. I like to refer to the "pillars of wellness" when discussing the healthcare journey. These eight pillars all impact our well-being.

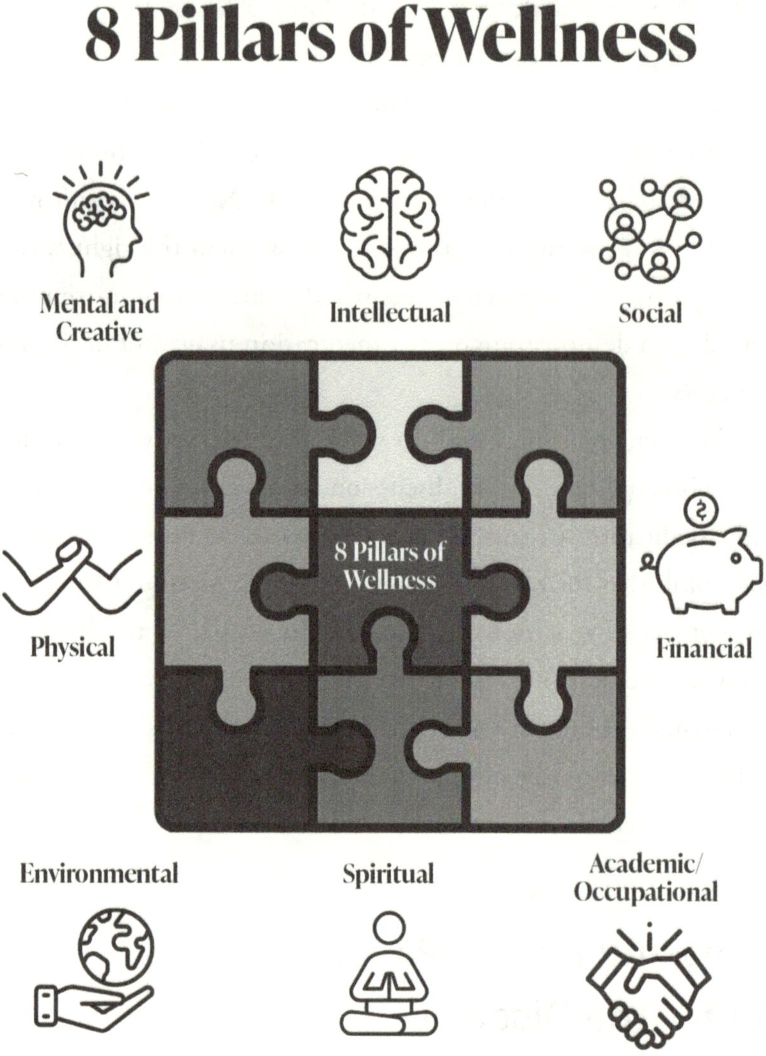

Figure 6.1: The eight pillars of well-being.

It's not just the medical diagnosis that matters. The whole patient matters—including these eight pillars, from environmental to occupational, spiritual, and beyond. For example, exposure to air pollution—an environmental pillar—can exacerbate asthma risk. This can come down to where a person lives or the type of work they do—an occupational pillar. In addition, a person may be living with more than one medical diagnosis or other complicating variables that require personalized consideration—physical pillars.

This well-rounded approach puts the person back into *person-*alized care, looking beyond the disease alone—which is essential if we are going to treat patients optimally. This personalization is especially critical in a disease such as asthma, which can vary significantly in severity and even fluctuate in a single individual over time. The Clinical Asthma Score and the Asthma Severity Score are two scoring systems used to help determine a patient's needs. Such asthma severity indices comprise various data points, including lung function, medication needs, and symptom burden. There is also the Asthma Control Test™, which provides a numerical score to assess asthma control. This is the kind of assessment that a physician may have a patient with asthma do to re-evaluate stability of symptom control over time.

However, a person can have more than one diagnosis, and although specific scales by disease state may be informative, they may lack important individual contributing factors. This is why I frequently recommend the use of a symptom diary—a printable version of which is linked to at the end of chapter 4. A symptom diary can be used in any medical situation and allows a person to record their lived experience across twenty-four hours, for one to two weeks at a time. Recorded features can include sleep schedules, eating patterns, symptoms experienced, factors identified to resolve or bring on these symptoms, and more. A symptom diary can be helpful in better capturing and understanding the burden experienced or improvements seen over time. This is because it illustrates the *lived* experience and, as such, may identify factors that seem unrelated but are contributory, actionable, and informative.

This collaborative effort can help augment self-efficacy by improving self-awareness and self-management, allowing a person to identify patterns and trends, lifestyle and behavioral contributors, adherence barriers, and triggers for worsening symptoms. Furthermore, it also facilitates improved communication between the patient and the healthcare system, and it better informs the development of an individualized assessment and plan by incorporating the right care, with the right team members, at the right time.

At this point, I am sure you recognize that the whole picture goes beyond the identified diagnosis. And, in Jonas's case, this is where Dr. Nelson has hit a wall. Dr. Nelson is treating the medical diagnosis: asthma. He sees an asthma patient—not Jonas, a person living with asthma. Starting with a person-first mindset helps limit the possibility of missing less obvious factors, such as socioeconomic status, cultural differences, or health literacy. In this case, Dr. Nelson is planning on treating Jonas as a person with a higher severity of asthma than Jonas actually has because he's failed to recognize the financial hurdles Jonas faces in adhering to treatment.

Unfortunately, individuals with a lower socioeconomic status are higher risk for asthma treatment failure and asthma exacerbations, including ICU admissions.[39] Not having insurance that pays for the medication is just part of the problem. Income impacts other factors, too, such as the patient's environment. For example, pests such as cockroaches have been shown to be a problem in some federally subsidized housing intended for low-income individuals, and cockroaches can exacerbate asthma.[40]

Communication Callout: Socioeconomics

It's no secret that socioeconomic status (SES) can impact health. Differences in SES can result in variations in living conditions, food choices, exposure to adverse childhood events, and even safety concerns. Healthcare considerations that can be relevant to SES include differences in access to care, insurance coverage, and health literacy. To further the point that SES impacts health and outcomes, there is evidence that correlates a person's zip code with how long they will live.[41] Change begins with systems that incorporate SES considerations in the establishment of community resources, recognizing access needs and developing tools to improve equity not only during but also between healthcare visits. The implementation of school-based partnerships, community activities with peer mentorship, and purposeful inquiry without stigma are the responsibility of all stakeholders to deliver on consistently. Awareness is the first step in changing these statistics. SES should not impact health outcomes. Period.

Adherence difficulties or lack of success with a treatment frequently result in a person being called a "treatment failure," creating stigma. However, that "failure" is often a reflection of a suboptimal healthcare system. Just because a medical diagnosis has been successfully made and a care plan implemented with a strategy that historically has been *medically* successful does not mean it's going to be successful *for that person.* For example, a person with persistent asthma is prescribed an inhaled oral steroid to reduce inflammation and swelling in the airways, but they are not given the anticipatory guidance to rinse their mouth after use. An inhaled oral steroid can create an oral environment that is prime for a yeast infection in the mouth called thrush. A person who experiences this may stop taking the medication as a result. They did not fail. Communication did!

Each of the eight pillars of wellness—from nutrition and exercise to finances and environment—plays a role in a person's overall health. By considering how these pillars interact with and influence a patient's condition, we can develop a more comprehensive understanding of their health status. For instance, poor sleep might exacerbate asthma symptoms, while proper nutrition could help manage inflammation. As HCPs, it's our job to connect these dots and see the bigger picture of our patients' lives, not just the isolated symptoms they present with.

What the **** Is Going On!?

This is the question that both the HCP and the patient are hoping to answer in the assessment and available option discussion. The HCP has been trained to quickly and efficiently give the most likely cause and the best plan of action. Frequently, the patient wants to know, "Doc, what the **** is happening to me?! What else do I need to worry about? And how do we make it go away?" As an HCP, this is where it is necessary to articulate how what was communicated during history-taking and found during the examination have been synthesized—and, based on the differential diagnoses, what steps you would suggest for either testing, treatment, or both. For those in the patient's seat, it is critical to convey what you understand and what you may need further clarity on.

In medicine, we falsely prepare clinicians to think that they have to have the correct answer the first time, every time. I've said it before, and I'll say it again: Time can be one of the greatest diagnostic tools. That said, a clear and confident discussion regarding what the next steps are and how the ongoing partnership will look, complete with defined roles and responsibilities on each side—plus identification of reasons for any potential detour—will bolster the likelihood of taking the correct path together.

Clarity is key. Ask yourself the right assessment questions to make sure communication is correct. It's important to discuss the diagnosis and its implications, cover treatments available (pharmaceutical, lifestyle, behavioral), and highlight social support resources as needed. HCPs must also prepare the patient for worst-case scenarios; don't sugarcoat. For example, we saw that Dr. Nelson had warned Jonas about the red flags that scream, "Go to the ER, now!"

ASSESSMENT QUESTIONS FOR HCPS TO ASK THEMSELVES

- Did I provide a summary of how the information the patient provided and the examination I performed informed me in forming my initial assessment?
- If I don't have a complete explanation right now, have I explained why and what other information is needed for better direction?
- Have I discussed the next steps and why they are necessary (e.g., tests or treatments)?
- When discussing treatments, have I shared what options exist and what my suggestions for treatment are based on right now?
- Have I provided anticipatory guidance on time to treatment response, possible side effects, medication interactions, and reasons to immediately discontinue if a severe adverse event occurs?
- Have I provided guidance on when to update me and when to follow up in person or via telemedicine?
- Have I introduced the role of other providers I work with and how they may interact with the patient as part of team-based care?

- Are there additional resources for education, social support, or other assistance that I can connect the patient to?
- Has the patient confirmed that they feel comfortable with the information and the plan?

From the patient's side, know that it's *always* OK to keep asking questions. Is the assessment aligned with what you are expecting? If not, does it make sense—has the HCP explained it to you in a way you understand? If you are given a concrete diagnosis and a care plan, does it all make sense to you?

ASSESSMENT QUESTIONS FOR PATIENTS TO ASK HCPS

- What's my diagnosis? And what should I expect with this diagnosis?
- Are further tests needed? If so, what should I expect in terms of these tests and time to receive results, and how will this impact my care?
- Are any alternative diagnoses possible?
- Are there specific symptoms I should record or monitor for?
- What treatment options are available? With these treatments, which are best when also considering my personal status (such as age, gender, reproductive status, comorbidity, other medications).
- Do I need to see a specialist? If so, what recommendations do you have on who I should see, and in what time frame should I be seen?
- What resources can you recommend for me to better understand diagnosis, testing, lived experiences shared by others, medications, or anything else I am not considering?

I've included links to printable versions of these checklists at the chapter's conclusion. The aim of these tools is to promote clarity and increase patient involvement. Again, we always want to keep the patient in the driver's seat! For this to happen, patients need knowledge—on their terms, in language that means something to them.

Qualitative research has shown that explanation of diagnostic evidence is a factor in patient involvement. Although these results come from a study specifically of oncology consultations, the findings may be transferable to other clinical contexts.[42] The results show that invoking diagnostic evidence, when appropriate, is an effective way of increasing levels of patient question-asking—which ensures that patients have the means at their disposal to determine their information needs. Basically, question-asking can bridge the gap between the doctor knowing what the **** is going on and the patient knowing what the **** is going on.

HCPs should further encourage patients to use tools outside the clinic to increase patient education, engagement, activation, and empowerment. Although research shows that physicians remain skeptical of Dr. Google—a term used to refer to the act of obtaining health information online[43]—there are high-quality, reliable resources available. Online resources can be one way to address the health literacy gaps that can otherwise impede the healthcare journey. The internet opens a wealth of resources appropriate to different languages, cultures, and contexts. A diversity of media is also needed to bridge the gap. Pages of written material full of medical speak aren't going to be useful for a patient with a fourth-grade reading level. Videos and graphics are a good alternative. These resources keep the patient in the driver's seat.

I've already discussed how a symptom diary provides a personalized look at an individual's current state in their healthcare journey. A complementary resource that can be developed based on the symptom diary is a progress map. A progress map outlines the patient's journey to an end goal—a desired outcome, such as "sleeping without snoring," "no longer feeling tired during the day," or "not experiencing pain when I do XYZ." By starting with the patient's desired outcomes and building from there, the progress map underpins patient-directed care. This is something I introduce regularly with my patients so we can see what is and isn't working for them over time. The progress map is also a reminder of the desired end destination, addressing the question, "What does progress look like?" For a patient with asthma, for instance, maybe it's being able to exercise regularly. The progress map sets expectations and reinforces accountability as the medical journey is navigated.

In Figure 6.2, we see what a progress map might look like for Jonas according to the chapter's opening narrative. Ideally, his trajectory would follow the horizontal arrow from diagnosis to final destination. But the reality of the healthcare journey is more complicated than that. We can see where the journey deviates from the desired path. That said, it's not all bad! We also see the progress. Jonas *is* moving toward his final goal.

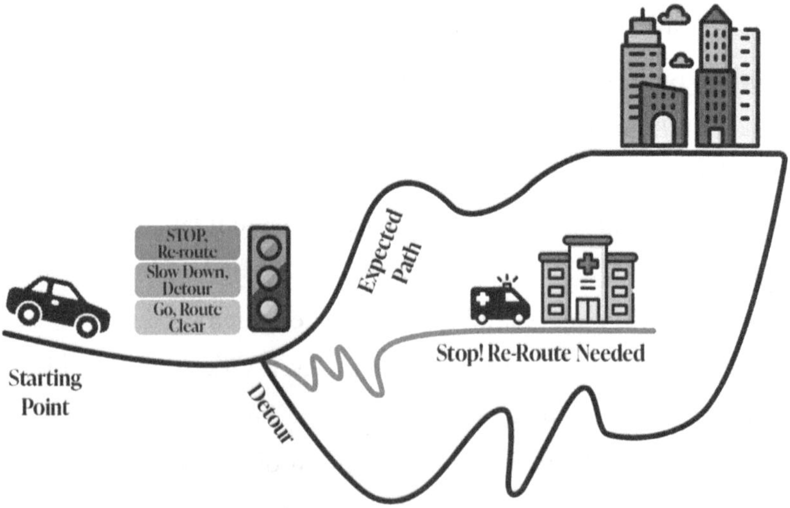

Figure 6.2: A sample patient progress map.

Progress Mapping Steps	Name It!	Expectations, Goals and Timelines
Starting Point/ Destination	**Specific disease or symptom targeted:** Poorly controlled asthma **Desired outcome:** Well-controlled asthma with improved wellness security in order to improve work function, socialization, and mental health	**Personalized impact from disease or symptom:** Frequent ER visits per month; multiple missed days or lateness to work; frequent albuterol use 3-4 times a day most days; reduced socialization due to not feeling well enough; weight gain because of not being able to work out and choosing foods that are inexpensive and pre-made due to lack of daily symptom predictability and fear of asthma attack; increasing anxiety about need for ER; losing employment; worsening depressed feelings about weight gain and reduced socialization
Choosing a Route	**Options listed singularly or in combination:** • Taking a daily controller medication • Short course of steroids • Or both	**Pros and cons of each option; relevance to personalized impact, goals, other health or wellness factors:** Pros: • Daily controller medication will help gain control of asthma (and life) • Steroids provide immediate asthma control to overcome current exacerbation alone • Reduced albuterol use Cons: • Potential difficulty in obtaining medication • Steroid side effects
Being Proactive	**Treatment-specific benefits; personalized value or impact; team players involved; behavioral and lifestyle factors to consider or implement; roles and responsibilities; potential risks and likelihood based on unique person profile:** • Over the course of this week, with the use of an oral steroid and inhaled controller, the need to use albuterol should be reduced to stopped completely. • Steroids will likely provide a more immediate impact to asthma control which will help reduce albuterol use and potentially improve response to controller medication. • The controller medication should be taken one puff with a spacer twice a day. The spacer provides a more effective delivery of the medication to your lungs. Rinse your mouth with water and spit after use to avoid a yeast infection in the mouth.	**Time to improvement and what that will look like; timing of possible side effects and how they may be experienced:** • Today you should not have chest tightness or shortness of breath at rest. You should have reduced to complete cessation of cough and shortness of breath with activity between today and 3 days with continued use. • During the period of taking steroids you may experience an impact on hunger, mental health, heart rate, blood pressure, blood sugar, and sleep. If this, occurs we can evaluate the need to stop the steroid.

Confirm Check-Ins	**Expected asynchronous and synchronous check-ins:** • MyChart messaging • Follow-up appointment **Unexpected or unscheduled events:** • Emergency room visit • Unscheduled office call or visit	**Specific times and types of interactions outlined; what should be monitored and communicated with each check-in** • Send a MyChart message to our team within 5-7 days to share with me your ability to obtain the medication prescribed, ability to use as directed, your perceived benefit, and any concerns of side effects. Please keep track of your ability to increase activity, attend work, improve socialization, and any changes experienced in mental health. • Schedule a follow up appointment in 4 weeks for re-evaluation. **What prompts an unexpected event and what actions should be taken:** Reasons to seek unscheduled care (need to re-route): 1. **Immediately by an emergency room:** • Breathing is hard and fast • Difficulty speaking due to breathing difficulty • Mental health crisis—feelings of self-harm or suicide; call 988 or go to your nearest ER 2. **With my office:** • Unable to obtain medication due to need for prior authorization, cost, or need for alternate type to be covered by insurance • Continued or escalating use of albuterol; persistent or worsening of symptoms; not responding to medication as expected • Concern of tongue whiteness or features of oral infection • Concern of side effects

**Note: Progress maps can change over time. However, rationale for change should be communicated and understood by all involved as well as documented in the record for recall to best personalize future mapping.*

The route taken in each patient journey may differ. However, the course becomes clear with a progress map. It's rarely, if ever, going to be a straight line from A to B! Unanticipated detours like Jonas experienced typically suggest that more information may be needed, indicating that we may be on the wrong course because something has changed or been challenged.

A NARRATIVE CASE STUDY, REIMAGINED

In the opening anecdote, Dr. Nelson confirmed that Jonas was able to report on how he should be taking his medication. However, both Jonas and Dr. Nelson checked Jonas's ability to demonstrate usage as prescribed essentially by reciting instructions. What about other common human factors that can lead to poor adherence? Let's see what happens when the patient's lived experience is considered.

I've really got to get out of here and get to work. But I don't want to end up in the ER again in a week. And Dr. Nelson seems like he really wants to figure out what's up with me.

"Let me just check my chart here and confirm your medications," he says as he looks at his tablet. "How are you doing with your new medication—any challenges with taking it?"

"No, I actually have them with me, like you said I should if I come to the hospital. The inhalers and the aerochamber. I use them every day," Jonas responds.

Dr. Nelson lights up and enthusiastically responds, "That's great. If you don't mind, can you show me how you use the medications so I can be sure we didn't miss any steps in teaching you how to take them most successfully?"

I show him how I use the inhaler, and Dr. Nelson nods approvingly.

Dr. Nelson takes the inhalers and looks on the back of them. He appears concerned and asks, "Jonas, can I ask you a question?"

Uh oh. I nod. But my stomach is flip-flopping. Why does the doc look worried?

"I notice that there are more treatments left in this inhaler than there should be, given the date it was prescribed. Some of my patients sometimes have difficulties taking medications multiple times a day and may miss doses. Other times, patients are concerned that they are taking too much medication. Or there may be other challenges to them taking their meds. Please don't take my question as judgment—I want to work with you to keep you well. Are you having any challenges with your meds?"

***

Jonas' face goes from fear to relief as he responds: "I was embarrassed to tell you that I try to stretch out the use because I still have a really high out-of-pocket expense for this medication, and I really can't afford paying that monthly until I meet my deductible." He then jokingly adds, "But I guess I can't really afford missing so much work, or all these ER visits, either."

I smile, grateful for his honesty. "I appreciate you sharing your challenge. This is actually great news, because we can change this. I have another option for a medication that we can use, and I will get our social worker to support with anything else that may be helpful. How does that sound?"

"That sounds good to me, Doc." Jonas looks visibly calmer.

"Good. I want you to follow up with your primary care physician in one week to check in on how you are doing. My goal, although I like you, Jonas, is to see you here a lot less."

Jonas grins but nods in agreement. Hopefully, I won't see him in the ER again anytime soon.

Jonas's journey had a bit of a detour but is now back on track. Just like the GPS in someone's car, the HCP-GPS can't get you to where you need to be if it doesn't know when you need to re-route. In the healthcare journey, identifying unanticipated barriers and providing timely redirection can get patients to their destination safely. Although we can't change systemic challenges that can be perceived as unfair barriers, we can fully address things within our control, such as alternative treatment strategies and improved self-efficacy, and still get to a life less burdened by symptoms.

COMMUNITY SUPPORT

More than twenty-five million people in the US live with asthma. Some races experience asthma at higher rates, including Black Americans, Native Americans, and certain Hispanic/Latino groups, particularly Puerto Ricans.[44] These organizations provide valuable resources for all: the **Allergy and Asthma Network**, the **Asthma and Allergy Foundation of America**, and the **Respiratory Health Association**. I have provided links to their websites in Appendix B.

Tests are frequently ordered with the intention of clarifying a diagnosis or perhaps even determining a response to treatment. However, what is frequently underestimated is the importance of communicating why a test is being ordered, what information it will provide, and how it will impact the ongoing care journey. Although this may seem obvious, communication and trust patterns that have already been established between the HCP and the patient become critical at this crossroads, as you'll see in the next chapter.

Growth Opportunity: Assessing the *Whole* Patient

In this chapter, I touched on some questions that HCPs can asks themselves—and that patients can ask HCPs—to bring clarity to the assessment and outcomes discussion. More comprehensive questionnaires that you can print off and use for yourself are available via the QR code.

Chapter 6 Endnotes

39 Torie Grant, Emily Croce, and Elizabeth C. Matsui, "Asthma and the Social Determinants of Health," *CME Review* 128, no. 1 (2022): 5–11, https://doi.org/10.1016/j.anai.2021.10.002.

40 Tom Neltner and Kathy Seikel, "Pests Persist in Federally Subsidized Housing," National Center for Healthy Housing and US Environmental Protection Agency, accessed December 4, 2024, https://nchh.org/resource-library/Case_Study_Conditions_10-14-07.pdf.

41 Jamie Ducharme and Elijah Wolfson, "Your Zip Code Might Determine How Long You Live—and the Difference Could Be Decades," *Time*, June 17, 2019, https://time.com/5608268/zip-code-health/.

42 G. M. Murtagh, L. Furber, and A. L. Thomas, "Patient-Initiated Questions: How Can Doctors Encourage Them and Improve the Consultation Process? A Qualitative Study," *BMJ Open* 3, no. 10 (2013): e003112, https://doi.org/10.1136/bmjopen-2013-003112.

43 Joanna Burzyńska, Anna Bartosiewicz, and Paweł Januszewicz, "Dr. Google: Physicians—the Web—Patients Triangle: Digital Skills and

Attitudes Towards e-Health Solutions Among Physicians in South Eastern Poland—a Cross-Sectional Study in a Pre-COVID-19 Era," *International Journal of Environmental Research and Public Health* 20, no. 2 (2023): 978, https://doi.org/10.3390/ijerph20020978.

44 "What is Asthma?" Allergy & Asthma Network, accessed December 4, 2024, https://allergyasthmanetwork.org/what-is-asthma/.

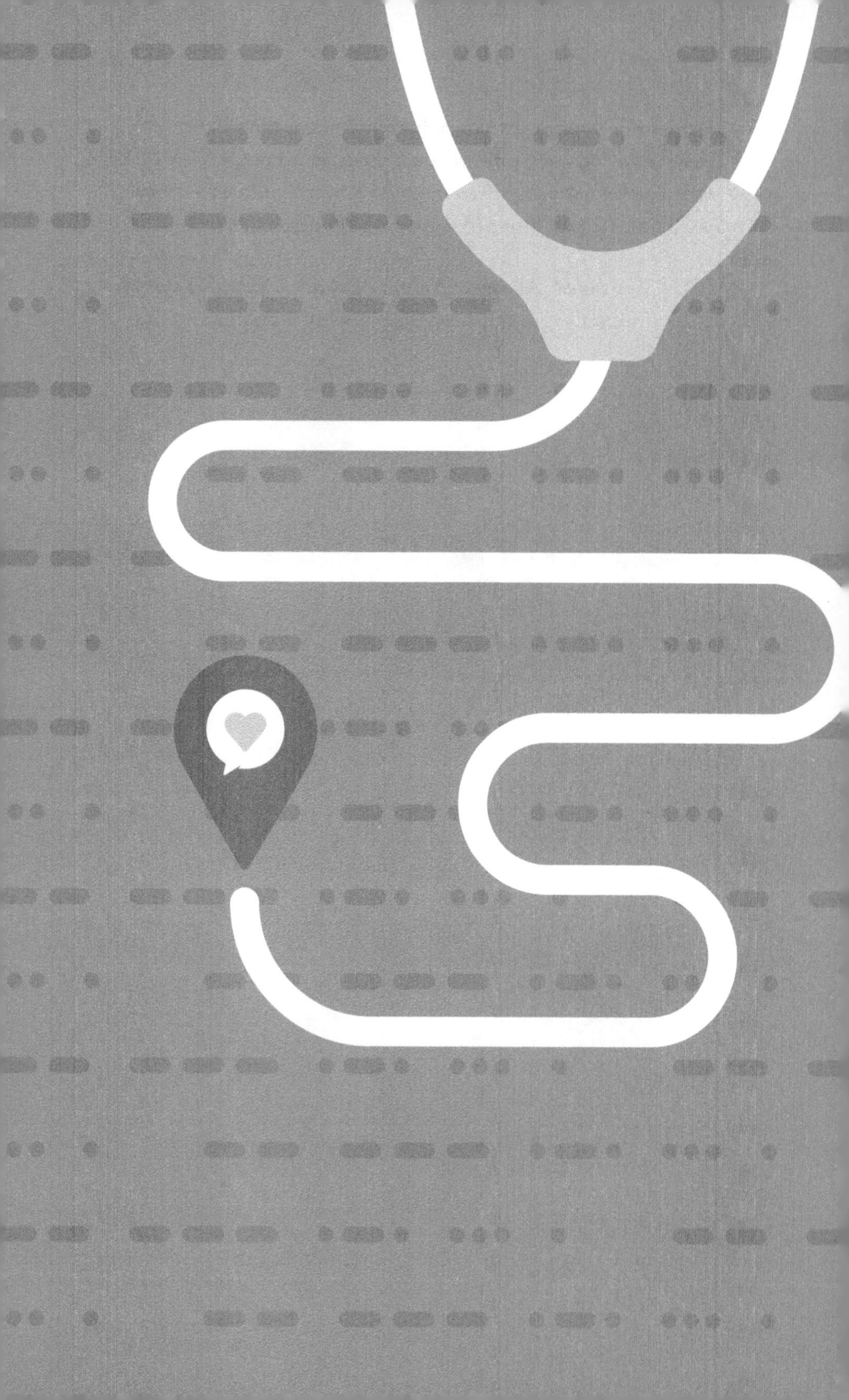

CHAPTER 7

Tests and Their Outcomes

The purpose of this chapter is to serve as a reminder of the role of tests and how to communicate their relevance. In most cases, histories and exams have already established the likely diagnosis. Tests, when needed, serve as the support for the most likely diagnosis.

NARRATIVE CASE STUDY: A PATIENT WITH A RARE DISEASE GETS TEST RESULTS

Zoe is a nineteen-year-old woman with Ehlers–Danlos syndrome, a group of inherited disorders that affect the body's connective tissues, from the joints to the skin and blood vessels. Up until now, Zoe has not been diagnosed, despite multiple clinical visits for issues related to the diagnosis. Dr. Bailey is going to help her get on the right path on her healthcare journey with an appropriate diagnosis, backed by the right test.

I can't believe I've dislocated my shoulder *again*! My mom says I'm clumsy. But I'm wondering if there's something else going on, so I'm seeing Dr. Bailey.

"So, Zoe, tell me what your concern is today?" The doctor fixes a friendly smile on me. "I understand you're recovering from a dislocated shoulder?"

"Yes, and it's the fourth time I've dislocated it."

The doctor sits up, looking more alert. "What were you doing when it happened? This time and in the past? Playing a sport?"

"One time, I was playing basketball with my brother. Then there was the time I fell while roller skating. Then I bumped into someone while walking. This time I wasn't doing anything strenuous—it was like I just leaned on my arm the wrong way. It was really weird."

"That *is* weird." Dr. Bailey nods. "I'm glad you came to me. Are you generally a very flexible person?"

"Yes, I guess so. I could always do a split."

"And do you ever have joint pain?"

"Yeah." I squint at the doctor, wondering what she's thinking. Finally, she reveals her thoughts: "Zoe, the reason I'm asking is that I'm wondering if you might have a genetic disorder. Have you heard of Ehlers-Danlos syndrome?"

"No." Suddenly, I'm scared.

"It's a genetic disorder that can include symptoms like overly flexible joints. Based on your history and the exam we just completed, I have a concern for this diagnosis, and I'd like to send you for testing to see if this might be what you're experiencing."

***

When people learn about an illness they've never heard of before, they're usually wondering if it's going to be some kind of death sentence. Most types of Ehlers-Danlos syndrome do ***not*** affect or lower life expectancy, which I make clear.

I help Zoe set up the test appointment, but I can tell that she is worried, so I give her some preliminary information about Ehlers-Danlos up front to reassure her. Since I suspect she'll go home and google it anyway, even without the diagnosis, I may as well give her reliable resources.

Three weeks later, I'm reviewing Zoe's test results. It turns out she does have Ehlers-Danlos syndrome. I'm glad we've identified it early.

I see that my team has already called Zoe and shared the test results with her. Now I have to get her back in the office to discuss a care plan, including a referral to a specialist.

***

I hang up my phone, feeling confused and scared. The nurse from Dr. Bailey's office just gave me my test results. I *do* have Ehlers-Danlos syndrome. But what do I do now? My brain is a mess of worried thoughts.

Dr. Bailey gave me some resources when I left her office after our last appointment, and I saw that the disease is genetic. Does that mean my kids could have it, if I have kids? Will this prevent me from having kids? What does this mean for my day-to-day life? Will this get worse as I get older?

The nurse wanted to make a follow-up appointment for me, but I was too rattled on the phone to make one on the spot. Suddenly, with all these thoughts flooding my brain, even the task of making a follow-up appointment seems impossible.

Three weeks ago, I'd never even heard of this illness. And now I have it?!

Ehlers–Danlos syndrome (EDS) qualifies as a rare disease—in the US, this means that fewer than two hundred thousand people live with the condition (other geographic regions may define a rare disease differently). This might make it sound as though HCPs will never encounter rare diseases in their careers. However, there are more than seven thousand rare diseases, affecting an estimated twenty-five to thirty million Americans. Given that about one in ten people in the US have a rare disease, the odds that an HCP will encounter one aren't so slim after all.[45]

In medical school, the general advice is, if you hear hoofbeats, look for horses, not zebras. However, based on the statistics cited above, 10 percent of people may be living with a rare disease that is just going unrecognized. I no longer teach my students and residents what I was taught (if you hear hoofbeats, think horses). Instead, I say, "Don't miss the dazzle [the term for a group of zebras] among the horses."

When the history and exam lead you to identify features that need more information to best clarify the diagnosis, testing may be necessary. In some instances, the right tests can play a valuable role in identifying rare diseases. In others, there is no definitive test for the disease. The first step is knowing *what* to test for—and this is where Dr. Bailey shines. With that stated, the doctor could improve her communication around the anticipatory guidance regarding what the test looks for, in describing how a positive result may impact Zoe's care, and in sharing the actual test result. A nurse providing test results and attempting to schedule a follow-up is a commonly encountered practice that is within the scope of normal procedures because it is efficient. However, it may fail to acknowledge that, for the patient on the receiving end, this represents a major detour—even a breakdown—in their medical journey.

I recall being a high school student when my oldest sibling received a call to say that her test results were back—she had lupus. She politely thanked the staff for the results but had no idea what this disorder was or what it meant for her. She then called my mother and my grandmother and asked if they had heard of it. My grandmother immediately began to cry and pray, as she recalled her brother who had passed away, aged fifteen, because of complications related to lupus. Although the test results confirmed the diagnosis, both my sister and my grandmother were lacking information. My sister was not aware of how serious lupus complications could be. Meanwhile, my grandmother had seen the effects lupus could have—albeit decades earlier, before treatment had improved. The gaps in my sister's story were then filled with each person's own interpretation of the information they did have.

Similarly, Zoe has been given a diagnosis without context. This usually goes in one of two directions—either the patient shrugs it off and there is a risk of them not following up, or they panic. Proactive steps can help regain control over the journey when the road is rough, with the HCP providing clinical guidance and/or the patient seeking information both when a test is ordered and after. The HCP, the patient, and the patient support system all need to actively engage in a discussion on why the test has been ordered, how it will be performed, the typical time to results, how the test will help the patient's course (whether it is positive or negative), and what the next steps will look like in a patient-directed care plan. This is exactly what Zoe needs, too, and at the end of this chapter, we'll see what her situation could look like if she gets it.

Getting the Most out of Tests

HCPs not only need to consider what to test for—they must also ask themselves what information a test will and will not tell them. It's necessary to consider what differentials can and can't be excluded based on a given test and with what certainty. Test results carry either a high-positive predictive value or a high-negative predictive value. If it's a high-positive predictive value and the test result is positive, it's likely the individual has the disorder being tested for. If it's a high-negative predictive value and the test result is negative, it's unlikely the individual has the disorder being tested for.

Further, there's the need to consider the sensitivity of the test. In some cases, tests need to be run more than once. Take a condition such as epilepsy, for instance. In such cases, I will order an electroencephalogram (EEG) to characterize the electrical activity of the brain. This will help me to understand the risk of recurrence and to identify the localization of seizure onset. If the EEG results are abnormal, this *could* suggest an increased risk for epilepsy and recurrent seizures—but it also depends on the abnormality observed. A single, routine EEG can appear normal in 40 to 50 percent of people with epilepsy, with some studies suggesting up to 73 percent showing a modest sensitivity. But if I repeat the EEG, sensitivity increases, and a more sensitive scan can identify more than 90 percent of people who may have epilepsy.[46]

A lot of thought goes into what tests to run, why, and how often. And as always, there are systemic issues at play. Medical tests can be costly. What insurance needs to be navigated? Has it lapsed? Even if it's in good standing, will it cover the testing? Does the system have the capacity to run the test needed in a timely manner? For instance, an MRI may be quickly scheduled and performed in most locations, but an MRI with sedation may not be performed for months—and many centers do not have the capacity to offer it.

Time is another systemic consideration. The test first needs to be scheduled, but it often requires preauthorization by insurance, and then it needs to be performed successfully. Healthcare systems risk losing patients to other systems when the time to test is prolonged. Frequently, an empowered patient will seek out the location that can meet their needs the soonest, unless otherwise discussed with their HCP. Unfortunately, this can fragment care by delaying results to the ordering provider. In some cases, the patient may lose confidence in healthcare system A and move to healthcare system B, believing that it will provide a better patient experience.

In medical school, we may get a gold star for identifying the right test or outcome of a test associated with a disease process. An overlooked but equally important focus is the discussion around *why* the test is ordered, when to expect it to be performed, how it will be performed, and how the results may inform the direction of an individual's healthcare journey. This is a major driver of miscommunication and misdirection in the healthcare journey. When ordering a test, consider using a template alongside the test order to help answer important test-related questions. This helps to keep everyone moving forward together.

EXPLAINING TESTS: TOPICS FOR HCPS TO COVER

- What test are you recommending or ordering?
- What information does this test provide, both in general and then specifically related to the condition of concern?

- What is the expected patient experience of the test?
- Is any specific patient preparation required?
- When and where should the test be performed?
- How soon will the test results be available?
- How will the test results help inform next steps for the diagnosis or treatment plan?
- Are there any risks related to the test?

I have included a link to a more comprehensive, printable version of this checklist at the chapter's conclusion. The most important thing is to explain what you're testing, why, and what to expect. Let's reflect on Zoe's experience with testing. Although there is a discussion about the concern for EDS, there has been no discussion about what the next steps will look like after the results are returned or what implications these results will have on her care. Although Dr. Bailey does an exceptional job of identifying the right diagnosis of concern, ordering the correct test, and explaining that it is to help confirm the diagnosis of EDS, there are gaps in her anticipatory guidance and in the delivery of the results.

As the person on the medical journey, there may be times when either you are not on board with the testing or you are requesting testing that is not being ordered. In both scenarios, this may be due to less-than-optimal communication. An opportunity exists to gain clarity. An improved understanding of the information that is shaping the diagnosis and treatment, and clarification about how completing or not completing specific testing is relevant, allows for transparency and security as the journey progresses. It is critical to take part in confirming that you understand and agree with the route being recommended—or not. This may require you to ask questions. If an HCP is going to request a test, you need to know what it's for. Alternatively, if there is a test you are hoping for and it's not being recommended, have a conversation about why. These questions can help you discuss testing in a way that is relevant to your specific situation.

UNDERSTANDING TESTS: QUESTIONS FOR PATIENTS TO ASK

- What's the purpose of the test?
- Why do (or don't) I need it?
- Is there any special preparation for the test? And what should I expect during the test?
- What risks or side effects may occur with this test?
- How will I know if this is covered by my insurance and what it may cost me out of pocket? Is there an alternative if I can't afford it?
- How long will it take to get the results? And how will I be contacted about the results?
- How will this test influence my diagnosis or care?
- How do I get a copy of the results for my personal records? Will the results be visible in my health record application?
- Are there alternative or additional diagnostic tools (e.g., if the test is invasive)?

The QR code at the chapter's conclusion links to a printable version of this checklist. There are also practicalities to consider. When going for a test, are there guidelines on how to prepare? For example, if the patient is going to be sedated, they may need someone to pick them up and drop them off. Do piercings need to be removed? Is lotion or deodorant a no-no?

As a physician, I myself have experienced the "I didn't know any better" testing faux pas. I went to my first mammography straight from work—so, of course, I had deodorant on. Although I dutifully used the cleaner provided to wipe it off before the test, the result of my first mammography came with a question mark: It was unclear as to whether the spots seen were concerning or artifacts. In most such instances, these spots are artifacts. However, for me, this happened to come at a time when my mother had just been diagnosed with lung cancer. So, dismissing my own fears and angry at myself for wearing the deodorant, I spent the next six months waiting for my repeat test—leaving me in a grim purgatory in my journey.

When it comes to test prep, the healthcare team is critical. The ordering clinician is only part of the team that is going to give the step-by-step guide on how to prep for a test. In the best-case scenario, the patient experiences a well-oiled team that performs as beautifully as synchronized swimmers, providing a seamless delivery in terms of expectations and follow-ups. Unfortunately, the experience is usually more fragmented.

When it comes to communicating test results, processes vary. Some healthcare systems differentiate who delivers the news depending on the test results. If it's a negative result (the suspected illness is not present), an administrative person can deliver it, but if it's a positive result (an illness is confirmed), a clinician must provide the results or have an appointment scheduled. In the case of positive results that require a specialist's follow-up, there's the handoff to consider. When and how will this be relayed to the patient, and by whom? If you get a biopsy to check for cancer, and the next thing you know, an oncologist is calling you to discuss the result, that can be scary. You'll immediately assume you have cancer.

Then there is the process of delivering the message itself—in person, via telemedicine, over the phone, or through a chart message? In what language, dialect, or tone? The lexicon is also a consideration.

Are the results conveyed in nonmedical jargon? Health literacy is also important to think about. What educational materials, including multimedia, can be used to communicate the test results and their implications effectively? Videos? Graphics? Infographics?

Communication Callout: Modes of Communication

The means used to communicate test results can influence how they are received. As technology proliferates, there are more options than ever, and the medium can make a difference. For instance, research suggests that communicating negative test results over text message can reduce patient anxiety.[47] However, face-to-face communication, whether in person or over video, allows the deliverer to pick up on body language clues that might otherwise be missed.

Finally, any communication of test results should include some sort of opportunity for follow-up or additional information. People who are receiving test results are usually digesting what they've just been told. They may not think of all their questions right away. Giving them an outlet to turn to for information when they're ready is essential.

Tests Provide Some—Not All—of the Answers

Even when test results are appropriately communicated, ambiguity sometimes remains. It's common to see confusion around the implications of test results. Just because you have the answers to a test doesn't mean you have *all* the answers.

Take genetic testing. The availability and use of genetic testing has exploded with the possibility of mapping entire genomes, and consumer products such as 23andMe are available for anyone to purchase. However, a genetic test alone does not present the entire clinical picture, and it can create unnecessary anxiety. A person can have a gene that may be considered a risk factor for a certain illness, such as cancer—however, the same individual can possess other traits, even other genes, that may confer protection *against* the development of cancer. Additionally, with ongoing scientific advancements, our understanding of genetics is changing, resulting in the possibility of gaps in the clinical picture. This concept is not unique to genetic testing; it can be applied to laboratory testing or imaging, where new concepts may improve and even replace prior diagnostic modalities, potentially resulting in a change in diagnosis.

Even when a test result can help confidently confirm a diagnosis, uncertainty can still linger, especially if the diagnosis has an unknown prognosis or there are limited to no recommended treatment options available. This can be especially true in the case of rare diseases. The diagnosis of a rare disease can introduce a unique challenge in that the diagnosed person may never have heard of it. The HCP who made the diagnosis may be equally unfamiliar. This lack of familiarity on both sides can contribute to a lack of trust based on fear of the unknown, resulting in both sides filling knowledge gaps in the story with less-than-optimal filler. This further underscores the critical importance of the point made throughout this book: of always leading with the foundational principles of trust, respect, communication, best-in-class care, and teamwork. Prior to the test, it's helpful to characterize any identifiable potential unknowns associated with a diagnosis of the rare disease—and to then connect the affected person to resources and a community that can support them and their knowledge-seeking on their journey. This is one of those times when an HCP should be able to say, "You know what, I've only read about this disorder in textbooks. Let's see what resources we can connect with so that both of us can gain more information."

Communication Callout: Social Listening

The greatest experts on any chronic condition tend to be those living with it, especially in the case of rare diseases. Understanding the lived experience with these conditions can better inform an understanding of the disorder's features, possible diagnostic considerations, and treatment strategies. The value is evident in the success of social listening, a data science in which novel disease concept maps are developed based on conversations with individuals living with specific medical conditions. TREND Community is one example. I have collaborated with this Philadelphia-based data analytics company for research and advocacy purposes, helping to turn the conversations of rare, chronic, and emerging disease communities into actionable insights. In one example, we explored the concept of "brain fog" in sleep disorders through a project entitled "Beyond Brain Fog: A Social Listening Analysis of Impaired Cognitive Functioning in Sleep Disorders."[48] To date, TREND Community has partnered with more than fifty patient communities spanning a range of disease states and symptoms, offering experience analysis and real-world evidence acceleration.[49]

Now let's look back to Zoe's experience of receiving an EDS diagnosis. In the opening version of her story, Zoe was given the results of her test over the phone and then left without a game plan. How might the pre-test anticipatory guidance and post-test communication be done differently?

A NARRATIVE CASE STUDY, REIMAGINED

Zoe was left to process her test results alone after receiving a phone call about her positive results and confirmed diagnosis from Dr. Bailey's nurse. What if Dr. Bailey had provided more anticipatory guidance and made the call herself—or even had the nurse better prepared to answer questions?

I strongly suspect Zoe has EDS. As I help her off the exam table, I steel myself for the discussion I'm about to have with her.

"Zoe, EDS is a genetic condition that causes a connective tissue disorder. Are you familiar with it?"

She shakes her head, already looking afraid.

"So, genetics are like the instructions for your body—how it should be made and how it should function. When a person has repeated experiences that don't match the expected development or function, that can suggest a genetic change—something about that person's 'instruction manual' is different."

"OK." Zoe nods slowly.

"Now, EDS is a connective tissue disorder characterized by problems with the tissues that hold the body together—commonly the parts that are made of collagen and elastin. These types of disorders can impact anywhere that connective tissues have a role, including the joints. There are times where the skin, eyes, heart, lungs, or GI system may be involved, too. Your history of repeated joint dislocations, along with findings from your exam, such as increased joint mobility and laxity or looseness of the skin, may indicate EDS. But I'd like to run a test to make sure. Before we do that, do you have any questions or concerns?"

Zoe shrugs, but she looks absolutely terrified. I place a reassuring hand on her shoulder. "Zoe, my intention is not to cause you fear, and I have the impression this is overwhelming to you to discuss. Can I make a suggestion?" Zoe nods, *yes*. "I am going to call our genetics counselor Jamie right now to introduce you. If there is a diagnosis of EDS—which we can't know for sure yet—she and I will be your co-pilots, helping you navigate life moving forward. I know it's scary, but getting this information will actually be helpful. We will be able to better predict and hopefully prevent future bumps in the road, like more dislocations."

Zoe's tension eases slightly, and she even manages a small smile. After I introduce Zoe to Jamie, we discuss the implications of a possible diagnosis with both Zoe and her parents. I then give her details about what to expect from her test and send her on her way with some links to EDS communities online.

A week later, Zoe's test results are back, and I see that she does have EDS. My team notifies patients of negative test results, but for this kind of positive result, I prefer to make the call myself. Before calling, I touch base with Jamie to reevaluate the plan we previously discussed with Zoe. Then I give Zoe a call.

***

When I see the number for the doctor's office on my phone's caller ID, I pick up right away. It's Dr. Bailey.

"Hi Zoe, its Dr. Bailey. I am reaching out because your test results came back today. Before calling you, I also called Jamie, the genetics counselor, to discuss the results with her to ensure we are all on the same page. The results do confirm the concern for the diagnosis of classical Ehlers-Danlos syndrome with an abnormality in a gene called *COL5A1*. This is the gene that gives instructions on making a part of your collagen."

"Yes, I remember discussing this with Jamie." I'm not thrilled by the news, but at least I sort of know what to expect. Jamie and Dr. Bailey already discussed potential care plans with me before the test–and I've been researching EDS online using the resources the doctor gave me.

Dr. Bailey speaks up: "What information can I provide right now about your diagnosis that will be helpful to you?"

"I guess I just want to know what happens next. I guess ... Do I need to see a specialist?" Dr. Bailey and Jamie had mentioned this already.

"Yes, I'd love to bring a specialist into your care plan to help us move ahead. How about scheduling a meeting to discuss next steps, and then I can provide the referral?"

I agree and immediately pull up my calendar on my phone. I want to see a specialist as soon as possible.

In this illustration, the value of team-based care is clearly illustrated. Dr. Bailey recognizes that Zoe has had much more opportunity to receive, digest, and even educate herself further on information about EDS. This has allowed her to be an active, empowered person, better able to partner with her care team in navigating her own care.

COMMUNITY SUPPORT

Frequently, the journey for many living with a rare disease is long, lonely, and laden with barriers to accurate diagnosis or treatment. The rare disease community is diverse, with numerous advocacy organizations and patient groups for different diseases. The **National Organization for Rare Disorders** is a centralized resource that represents all rare disease resources for patients, HCPs, researchers, and advocates. I've linked to this in Appendix B.

Tests can inform on the already suspected diagnosis, making them a valuable piece of the puzzle. However, they must be purposefully utilized in a balanced way, as there is also a risk that unnecessary testing can misdirect diagnosis and care. At the end of the day, patient partnership, optimal communication, and patient-directed care will keep the healthcare journey on track.

Growth Opportunity: Ready to Ace the Test?

In this chapter, I outlined some questions that HCPs and patients should consider when discussing tests. The QR code below will take you to expanded versions of these question lists: one for HCPs and one for patients. You can print these and use them.

Chapter 7 Endnotes

45 "Rare Disease Day: Frequently Asked Questions," National Organization for Rare Disorders, accessed December 4, 2024, https://rarediseases.org/wp-content/uploads/2019/01/RDD-FAQ-2019.pdf.

46 M. Salinsky, R. Kanter, and R. M. Dasheiff, "Effectiveness of Multiple EEGs in Supporting the Diagnosis of Epilepsy: An Operational Curve," *Epilepsia* 28, no. 4 (1987): 331–334, https://doi.org/10.1111/j.1528-1157.1987.tb03652.x.

47 Ipek Gurol-Urganci, Thyra de Jongh, Vlasta Vodopivec-Jamsek, Josip Car, and Rifat Atun, "Mobile Phone Messaging for Communicating Results of Medical Investigations," *Cochrane Database of Systematic Reviews* 6, (2012): CD007456, https://doi.org/10.1002/14651858.CD007456.pub2.

48 Maurice Flurie, Zachary Cline, Anne Marie Morse, Matthew Horsnell, Jennifer Gudeman, Lauryn Craine et al., "Beyond Brain Fog: A Social Listening Analysis of Impaired Cognitive Functioning in Sleep Disorders," paper presented at Sleep 2024, Houston, TX, June 1–5, 2024, https://trend.community/wp-content/uploads/2024/05/SLEEP_2024_QR_Code.pdf.

49 "How We Work," TREND Community, accessed December 4, 2024, https://trend.community/how-we-work.

CHAPTER 8

Patient-Directed Care

The purpose of this chapter is to provide guidance on how to set up a patient partnership for success. The healthcare journey is best navigated by having the patient in the driver's seat and the HCP as the trusted GPS. Medical care has transitioned from a paternalistic model to one that is now considered to be patient-centered, with a suggestion of shared decision-making. However, I believe that patient-centered care still conveys the idea of doing things *to* the patient, not *with* them. The concept of patient partnership presented throughout the book is based on patient-directed care, where the HCP and the person on the healthcare journey are on an equal footing, both contributing their relative expertise, resulting in an educated, active, and empowered patient.

NARRATIVE CASE STUDY: WHEN LIVING WITH OBSTRUCTIVE SLEEP APNEA COMPLICATES MORE THAN SLEEP

Jordan is a forty-year-old father of two. His wife has been complaining about his snoring. In fact, their sex life has taken a hit, as they are now sleeping in separate rooms. Even when the opportunity arises, Jordan struggles with performance. He assumes it's because of the snoring and lack of sleep, not realizing that erectile dysfunction can be related to obstructive sleep apnea (OSA). With the additional features of insomnia, he would have a diagnosis of comorbid insomnia and sleep apnea (COMISA), which comes with additional health risks. Jordan has several comorbidities, including diabetes, hypertension, and high cholesterol. He is meeting Dr. Sage, who has just given him his diagnosis.

I've just learned I have sleep apnea. My doctor explained that it's a special kind of sleep apnea that also comes with insomnia. Clarissa? No. Comissa. I think that's what she said. I snap back to attention, realizing Dr. Sage is still talking.

"So, now that we've got a diagnosis from your home sleep test, we can start figuring out some solutions."

"Great, because I'm tired of being tired all the dang time. And my wife is tired of my snoring." I don't add the fact that my snoring has also taken a toll in the bedroom in other ways. Our sex life is practically nonexistent—which sucks, because we want to have another baby!

"I bet," Dr. Sage nods. "And the good news is, there are a lot of solutions for sleep apnea."

The doctor shows me a machine that she says will help—a CPAP. It looks like it would be a pain to sleep with.

"Are there any other options?" I ask hesitantly.

"PAP therapies are the preferred therapy for OSA. It's usually the first line of treatment. If that doesn't work for you, we can explore alternatives," Dr. Sage says firmly. "So, I'd like to get you an autoPAP, which will be able to use a range of pressures to treat your sleep apnea. I'll have the request sent to a DME company. The team at the DME can outfit you with an appropriate mask that will be comfortable."

"Uh, sure ..." Now I'm confused. She said there are all these options. Why am I only hearing about one?

"I also want to refer you to a few specialists regarding some of the other test results based on your age, history, vital signs, exam, and recent labs. I'll send referrals to a cardiologist, a nutritionist, and an endocrinologist."

I nod, but I'm getting nervous. Why do I need to see all these experts? What does she mean about my age and all the other things? I am not that old. Am I sicker than Dr. Sage is letting on? I thought I just had trouble sleeping!

***

I notice the discomfort on Jordan's face, and I realize I've let myself get caught up in the medicine without explaining the ***why*** of what I'm saying. I take a beat.

"I know your primary concern was sleep problems. And we have identified that you have both insomnia and OSA, which is frequently referred to as COMISA. However, as part of your yearly physical, we discussed that your blood pressure and your body mass index were both elevated, placing your body profile as overweight, bordering obese. We also did some labs to check things like your cholesterol, blood counts, and blood sugar. Today, your blood pressure is again elevated. The labs also show an elevated cholesterol profile, and your hemoglobin A1c, a blood marker of blood sugar control, is elevated and consistent with a diagnosis of diabetes. COMISA can further aggravate your body's ability to control all these points, so I'd like to get the opinion of these specialists to best coordinate your care."

"OK," Jordan nods, understanding dawning on his face. Still, he looks overwhelmed. I can't blame him. The comorbidities that come with OSA can be a lot. But if I get a great care team on his side now, I'm confident we can get his health to where it needs to be.

"Are there any other symptoms we haven't discussed yet—or anything else that's worrying you?"

Jordan pauses. For a moment, I think he's going to say something. But he shakes his head.

"OK then, let's get your PAP ordered and these referrals ready."

Healthy sleep is a critical but commonly overlooked contributor to optimal health and wellness. Disturbances in the duration, timing, regularity, and quality of sleep or wakefulness are all potential findings of a sleep–wake disorder. OSA has been found to be an independent risk factor for many medical conditions, such as hypertension, diabetes, kidney disease, and atrial fibrillation. Jordan has developed multiple medical conditions and would benefit from a transdisciplinary approach. He needs care from several different specialists. Already, he is looking at a more complex patient journey than anticipated. Dr. Sage recognizes the complexity of his needs and is eager to connect Jordan with the appropriate specialists. She also explains why this is necessary. So far, so good.

However, we see a communication breakdown when it comes to the OSA treatment. Jordan is reluctant about CPAP and is left to wonder why he *must* try this option even though Dr. Sage alluded to other possible therapies. In general, positive airway pressure (PAP) has been considered the preferred and gold-standard treatment for sleep apnea for years. However, this doesn't mean it's preferred by patients.

This was crystallized clearly for me by one of my favorite people and sleep friend, Atul Malhotra. Atul is the epitome of expertise in sleep apnea. At a medical education event in which he and I participated, he reflected on a presentation he had given in which he had said exactly what Dr. Sage stated: "PAP is the preferred therapy for the treatment of OSA." During this presentation, he was asked, "Who prefers this therapy—you or the patient?" He told me that this changed his practice forever, making him realize he needed to consider the patient's preference. From that point forward, he has always made sure to present patients with all possibilities, which range from mandibular advancement devices to hypoglossal nerve stimulators.

With that stated, most patients will still have an experience like Jordan's and be offered PAP therapy first. If PAP is not a success, *then* the patient may be given other options (a generally accepted measurement of "success" or adherence to PAP use is relatively consistent use of, on average, at least four hours per night for at least five days per week). Unfortunately, many patients like Jordan will be deemed "PAP failures," which stigmatizes the individual and invalidates their efforts to participate in their own care.

The bigger failure lies on the side of the healthcare ecosystem. Because if the generally accepted patient adherence is not observed in the first three months, despite patient effort, insurance will revoke the equipment. Yes, you read that correctly: the individual is penalized by having their treatment taken away. And to make matters worse, the person will have to undergo another sleep test to *prove* that they still have sleep apnea *before* being eligible to try PAP therapy again.

Jordan's current stop on his journey illustrates why it's necessary to consider the whole person and their whole day. Dr. Sage has gotten off on the right foot by appropriately addressing the full twenty-four hours and offering an approach to treatment; but unfortunately, she has left Jordan vulnerable by not discussing all possible treatments that could improve the likelihood of patient adherence.

Finally, although the conversation between Jordan and Dr. Sage is relatively complete, Jordan decides not to include his concerns about sexual dysfunction. This may be related to his own perception that it's just caused by a behavior he needs to change, or it's possible he's embarrassed. We'll revisit this question when we return to the narrative case study at the end.

Communication Callout: "Taboo" Topics (Hint: There Are None)

HCPs learn to become comfortable with all kinds of topics—including anything sex-related. However, these may be topics that are considered "taboo" and which may not be broached by either the HCP or the person seeking care. Frequently, it becomes critical for the HCP to recognize medical associations with conditions such as sexual dysfunction. OSA is a perfect example: it is a well-known risk factor for erectile dysfunction. Even if a patient has not expressed a certain symptom, the HCP might present it as a possibility indirectly. For example, "OSA can have a lot of medical consequences you might not expect, including high blood pressure and erectile dysfunction." As for patients, remember that HCPs can't read your mind! Use your voice.

Whose Preferred Therapy—the Patient's or the HCP's?

As an advocate for a transformed healthcare ecosystem that prioritizes patient partnership and patient-directed care, I frequently reflect on the words used in healthcare. Terms such as "preferred therapy" epitomize the hurdles patients face. HCPs frequently use this terminology when referencing what are considered first-line therapies—but such therapies are not necessarily patient preference. In the same vein, we will also say that a patient has "failed" a treatment when the therapy prescribed fails to improve the symptoms or disorder it was intended for. The truth is that the system, not the patient, has failed by not providing adequately personalized care. If we hope to take the best course, we need to consider the *patient*-valued outcomes (note I did not say value-based outcomes [VBO]).

A patient-valued outcome is one that is a priority for the patient. If a planned strategy does not represent a person's concern or priority, how strict can you reasonably expect adherence to be? Throughout this book, we have seen how communication failure has many faces and contributors during all phases of the journey and how it impedes progress toward the desired destination of optimal outcomes. Fortunately, there is a large body of research that has explored adherence challenges and how they can present across individuals. Let's review these here:

- insufficient understanding around how and when to use a therapy
- lack of recognition of the therapy's benefits
- a desire to avoid unwanted side effects
- access hurdles
- affordability challenges

Take Jordan's case. Dr. Sage states that the good news is that there are multiple options, but she only presents one. In addition, there is no explanation of its prioritization, use, or benefit. Why is this the starting point? How will this first option help Jordan? When is it right to explore other options? This could be another lead-in point that Dr. Sage can use to address other problems that can occur with OSA, such as sexual dysfunction. What can both HCPs and patients do to get patient-directed care on track? When discussing therapies, it's all about the exchange of information.

DISCUSSING THERAPIES: POINTS FOR HCPS TO COVER

- What data supports the use and prioritization of this therapeutic option?
- What stats back this therapy's effectiveness?
- What possibility and types of adverse effects are there?
- When might adverse effects happen? Does anything make them more likely to occur?
- If applicable, how will this therapy be used concurrently with others?
- What future steps, including potential alternative therapies, are available?
- Has anticipatory guidance been covered? This includes time to effectiveness, alternative plans should adverse effects occur, reasons to book a non-planned appointment or seek emergency care, and, assuming things are going well, time to next appointment.
- What is the role of referrals, if applicable? Since certain therapies require an expert referral, this may be inevitable.

As we saw in the previous chapter, HCPs must also consider and articulate accessibility issues, such as potential costs or prior authorization needs, when discussing a therapy. This raises some big-picture considerations. What insurance does the patient have? Is this therapy covered? If not, is there something similar that *is* covered? People may label these things as frustrating. However, I encourage abandoning the use of the word "frustrated." By definition, it indicates a response to something you can't influence or change. And the whole point of this book is to emphasize what we can control and change. Familiarity with typical barriers empowers, helping to improve the likelihood of insurance approvals. Patients can also take steps to diminish their potential vulnerability and take control.

DISCUSSING THERAPIES: QUESTIONS FOR PATIENTS TO ASK

- What are the advantages of this therapy for my diagnosis?
- Are there alternatives?
- What is the likelihood this will help me?
- How soon will I experience the benefit?
- What are the possible side effects? When might they occur?
- Can I use this therapy safely with other medicines/therapies/treatments? (Tell your HCP about everything you take, including herbal/natural supplements.)
- What if this therapy doesn't work for me? Are there other options?
- What is the end destination you want to put into your GPS—is this therapy going to help you get there?
- Communicate any concerns you have about the potential strategy. Restate your priorities.

It is imperative to advocate for yourself when discussing therapies and to articulate what matters. The HCP cannot (and should not) assume the patient's goals. Patient-directed care requires the patient to set the path.

Assessing Therapies, Together: Symptom Diary and Progress Map

The need for HCP–patient communication doesn't stop once a therapy has been decided. When it comes to a question such as "How will we know if this therapy is working?", for example, both sides have a part to play. HCPs can know the medical requirements of what constitutes good adherence and efficacy. Patients can know the lived impact that a therapy has on them. This is where two tools we've discussed previously, the symptom diary and the progress map, can be useful.

Progress Mapping Steps	Name It!	Expectations, Goals and Timelines
Starting Point/ Destination	Specific disease or symptom targeted; desired outcome	Personalized impact from disease or symptom
Choosing a Route	Options listed singularly or in combination	Pros and cons of each option; relevance to personalized impact, goals, other heath or wellness factors
Being Proactive	Treatment specific benefits; personalized value or impact; team players involved; behavioral and lifestyle factors to consider or implement; roles and responsibilities; potential risks and likelihood based on unique person profile	Time to improvement and what that will look like; timing of possible side effects and how they may be experienced
Confirm Check In	Expected asynchronous and synchronous check ins; unexpected or unscheduled events	Specific times and types of interactions outlines; what should be monitored and communicated with each check in; what prompts an unexpected event and what actions should be taken

**Note: Progress maps can change over time. However, rationale for change should be communicated and understood by all involved as well as documented in the record for recall to best personalize future mapping.*

CREATING A PROGRESS MAP

1. Characterize and confirm starting place and desired destination
2. Jointly determine best route to take based on personal preferences and considerations (i.e. quickest, safest, more focused on one disease or symptoms, more comprehensive with multiple symptoms or diseases impacted, or a combination of factors)
3. Be Proactive: Lay out expected timeline and milestones of selected course, including:
    a. time and type of improvement,
    b. possible worsening or emergence of new symptoms,
    c. adverse events, and
    d. when relevant, potential impact on other medical or psychiatric factors to monitor and whether there are individual factors that may elevate risk.
5. Confirm check in points, reasons to signal for help or possible re-routing

When assessing therapies, the symptom diary can help to inform a progress map—something we first saw in chapter 6. Along with relevant medical tests, the progress map can help to determine how the patient's journey is progressing. It can also allow both the HCP and the patient to see what is and isn't working, not only from a medical perspective but also from a personal lifestyle viewpoint.

POINTS TO INCLUDE IN A PROGRESS MAP

Creating this map is a joint effort that requires honest discussion between the HCP and the patient. Points to include are:

- The patient's desired outcome/end destination
- The therapy that can help reach that end destination
    - What therapy?
    - Implemented at what date?
    - Conduct an adherence assessment
- Supporting lifestyle changes to help reach that end destination
    - What changes?
    - Implemented at what date?
    - Conduct an adherence assessment
- Timeline for reassessment, e.g., X days/weeks/months/years
- Setbacks on the journey, as evidenced by:
    - Symptoms diary
    - Medical tests
- Progress on the journey, as evidenced by:
    - Symptoms diary
    - Medical tests
- Deviations from the journey
    - Anything that takes the patient off the straight line to their end destination, e.g., adverse side effects, emergency room visits
- Reiteration or reconfiguration of the end destination/goal(s)

These tools are especially helpful when it comes to complex cases like Jordan's. If the patient has multiple comorbidities to track, treat, and manage, staying on top of it all is tricky. Compiling all relevant data in a single document helps to simplify matters and ensures a robust dataset that can be communicated easily to HCPs.

Progress maps can change over time. The solution you determine today isn't necessarily etched in stone. It can be revised—and nine times out of ten, it will be! The impetus for change could come from an HCP or a patient. Sometimes an HCP will suggest a shift because the efficacy isn't as expected. Sometimes a patient will suggest an alternative because a therapy isn't aligning with their lifestyle. In some cases, the map might change because of a new medical development, which can be suggested by a patient just as well as by an HCP.

With these tools, patient-directed care becomes a natural framework. However, even in patient-directed care, the HCP always has a medical duty of care. Patients can express desired outcomes and preferences regarding therapeutic treatments, but they must remember that doctors take the Hippocratic oath to do no harm. If a cancer patient tells their oncologist, "You know what, I don't want to deal with the side effects of chemo," that's their right. However, the oncologist can't just say, "OK, then!" If the oncologist has deemed that chemotherapy is necessary, they have a duty of care to impart this to the patient. Of course, you can't force someone into adherence. But you can't just bow to every whim and wish. "Do no harm" is the HCP's guiding principle.

Communication Callout: Culture and Religion

When considering therapeutic options, the implications of a patient's culture and religious beliefs may need to be taken into account. A patient needs to communicate how these may impact their consideration of certain therapies. HCPs must be aware of how to handle potential hurdles to care both ethically and legally. When feeling uncertain about challenging care considerations, the ethics teams at a healthcare institution can help navigate any rough waters. Appendix B includes a link to a useful primer from the **University of Pennsylvania Health System**, which explains how religious beliefs can impact patient decisions.

Ultimately, patient adherence starts with patient buy-in—and communication is the key to gaining it. Let's see how a more in-depth conversation between Dr. Sage and Jordan could get his care plan off on more secure footing.

A NARRATIVE CASE STUDY, REIMAGINED

When we left Jordan and Dr. Sage at the chapter's opening, Jordan was feeling overwhelmed by a diagnosis of OSA plus comorbidities. Let's see how Dr. Sage and Jordan might benefit from the two tools we've discussed—the symptom diary and the progress map.

I can see Jordan is having doubts about PAP therapy, so I do my best to explain why I'm recommending this as a first line of action.

"I know I mentioned some other therapies, Jordan, but PAP therapy is and has been used as an effective therapy for more than thirty years. It has been shown to effectively address the concerns you've voiced to me, such as daytime fatigue and snoring at night. It is also a treatment that will be important to help with the other medical concerns we have identified, like weight management, blood sugar control, and blood pressure."

"OK, I guess I'll give it a try."

"It would be really good if you did. However, I would like to review with you all the other considerations, so you are well-informed, but also in case you would like to consider a different route." As Jordan listens closely, I detail his other options, explaining how each one works. By the time I'm done, Jordan looks even more overwhelmed.

"That is a lot of options." He pauses, uncertain. "I think the CPAP sounds like a good place to start. But it's good to know there are other avenues to explore, too."

I smile. "I agree. It is good to have options and a game plan. Speaking of a game plan, ours will include us tracking your progress with the data the PAP itself records, such as how frequently you're using it, and also with a symptom diary."

"Like the one I used before?" Jordan looks confused. "I thought that was just to diagnose me."

"Well, it will be helpful in tracking how well the therapy is working for you going forward, too. And we will combine that feedback we get from you with metrics like blood glucose levels, blood pressure, and more, to make sure we're on the right course."

"OK."

"I'd also like to draw up a progress map for you. It will help us see how you're progressing toward your goal. So, let's start with exactly that: your end goal. What's your perfect outcome?"

"To stop being tired all the time," Jordan answers honestly. "And to stop snoring. It's driving my wife crazy. When it gets bad, she forces me to sleep on the couch–which isn't ideal, because we're trying for another baby," he adds with a shy smile.

"That's exciting!" I can see that Jordan looks a bit embarrassed at sharing this last detail–but I'm not fazed by it in the least. In fact, I'm glad he mentioned it. Because it reminds me that there's another side effect of OSA I haven't discussed with him yet: erectile dysfunction. "How long have you two been trying?"

"A few months now. Kind of. On and off. When I'm not too tired."

***

Dr. Sage nods–and then she says something that takes me by surprise. "Getting this OSA under control should hopefully give you all a hand. You know, OSA can also cause other problems, such as sexual dysfunction, including decreased desire and erectile dysfunction. Now that I know you want to start a family, that's even more reason to get you started on this therapy ASAP."

"That's good to know," I say, trying to hide my shock. I had no clue that my sleep problems could affect my sex life. Things have been fine, I think, but it's good to know. And now I'm even more sold on whatever solution Dr. Sage might have for me.

Here, Dr. Sage goes into more detail about Jordan's options to treat OSA and the *why* of the PAP therapy. She also articulates another possible consequence of OSA that makes Jordan take notice: erectile dysfunction! At the end, Jordan is left with more information, has confirmed his choice of preferred therapy, and is more motivated to give the therapy a try, which will improve his odds of adherence and, in turn, of reaching his end goal.

COMMUNITY SUPPORT

OSA impacts an estimated 39 million US adults.[50] Untreated, it can have dire consequences, such as impaired quality of life and functioning, adverse health outcomes, and impaired cognition and mood. Sleep is a tool for healthy living! Some resources for patients and HCPs alike (links in Appendix B) are available from the **American Academy of Sleep Medicine** and **DAMM Good Sleep**.

The healthcare journey is rarely linear. Tools such as a progress map can help delineate a path to success by defining what success looks like and providing clear anticipatory guidance on what the path to that final desired destination might entail. However, this doesn't guarantee that the journey won't have detours. For example, Jordan may have difficulty using the mask for his CPAP and may require additional guidance from Dr. Sage or the equipment company—or he may need to consider an alternative preferred therapy. Expectation-setting plus regular check-ins will help Jordan get back on track in the case of any such detours. Instead of looking in the rearview mirror at the turn we missed, let's keep our sights on the highway to health.

Growth Opportunity: Mapping Patient Progress

Creating a patient progress map is a team activity that requires the expertise of both the HCP and the patient. This is a living document that isn't just created once and set aside; it is referred to repeatedly and revised as needed, helping to track the patient's progress (and setbacks) on the way to the desired end goal. This template can serve as a starting point—scan the QR code for a version you can download.

Chapter 8 Endnotes

50 "Sleep Apnea Statistics and Facts You Should Know," National Council on Aging, October 9, 2024, https://www.ncoa.org/adviser/sleep/sleep-apnea-statistics/.

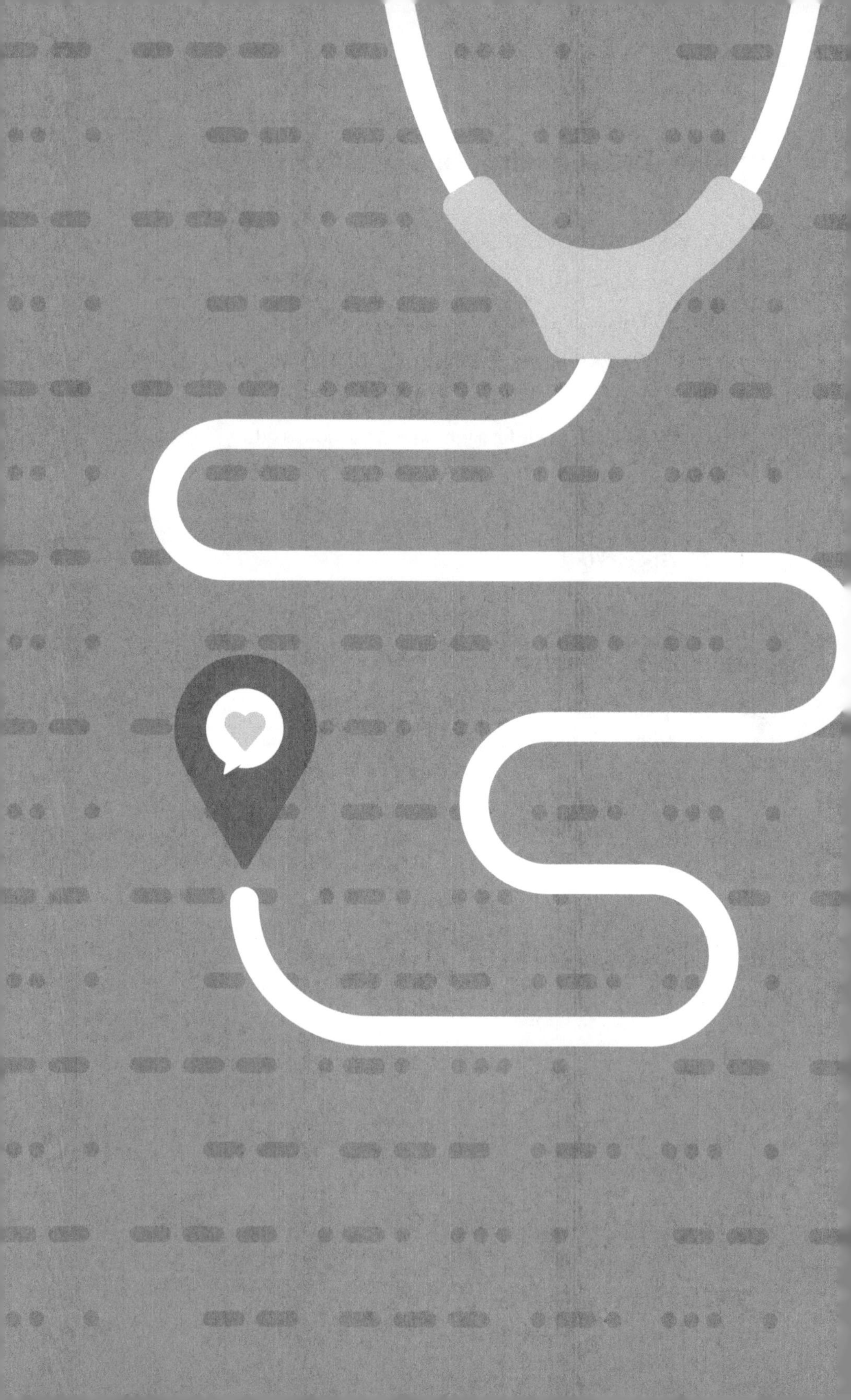

CHAPTER 9

Service Recovery

It's inevitable that some relationships will hit road bumps or blocks during the healthcare journey. When it comes to service recovery, or resolving the challenges experienced between the healthcare system and the person on their journey, great communication becomes even more essential. A negative experience can cause a loss of trust or confidence in the system, a poor outcome, or—as was the case for my mom—a loss of hope. This chapter looks at how we can heal those fractured relationships.

NARRATIVE CASE STUDY: PARENTS SEEK HELP FOR THEIR CHILD WITH A FUNCTIONAL DISORDER

Functional disorders are a group of disorders and syndromes characterized by recurring or chronic physical symptoms that are either disproportionate or unrelated to any biomedical pathology. Although the symptoms aren't rooted in any identifiable physiology, they may be severe enough that they cause some

level of functional impairment or disability. Here, our pediatric patient, Jonathan, aged fourteen, has been complaining of stomach pains. They are bad enough that he has missed several weeks of school. His concerned parents agreed to an endoscopy and a colonoscopy after multiple non-invasive tests did not reveal any identified pathology. Dr. Lee is giving them the results.

I smile as I deliver the good news to Jonathan's parents while Jonathan quietly plays a game on his phone. "Mr. and Mrs. Dennison, I've got good news. The endoscopy and colonoscopy for Jonathan were clear."

The parents sink back into their chairs, hands clasped, relief washing over them. I give them a moment to let it sink in before explaining further. "This allows us to rule out a few possible causes for his stomach and GI pains, including celiac and inflammatory bowel disease."

"That's great," Mr. Dennison replies, nodding.

However, Mrs. Dennison still looks concerned. "But he's still missing school." She shakes her head worriedly. "He's missed fifteen days in the last two months alone. And he's withdrawing from friends and avoiding eating!"

I keep my expression impassive, but I'm concerned. Jonathan's stomach pain may be a functional disorder without a physiological reason. However, based on what his mom is saying, not only is it a detriment to his day-to-day life, but it could also develop into a true medical problem, such as anorexia and malnutrition. But I don't want to scare these worried parents right now.

"Well, the good news is that Jonathan's still trending on the same weight curve. So, although he's experiencing a loss of appetite, he's maintaining a healthy weight for his age." First, I want to provide reassurance. But I also want to figure out how to help Jonathan.

"That's great news," Mr. Dennison cuts in. I see him place a calming hand on Mrs. Dennison's shoulder. She shrugs it off. Having a child who is not well can be tough on parents.

***

I can see that Dr. Lee is trying to keep us calm, but I can't stop the panic from rising in me. Meanwhile, my husband is acting like everything is great. I suppress an eye roll as I shrug his hand off me.

"So, how do we resolve what's happening?" I press on. I want answers for my kid! Jonathan seems fine now, happily playing Roblox on his phone, but I've seen him doubled over in pain, tears in his eyes, one too many days. "What can I do? You're telling me that physically he's fine. So, what, I just send him to school, even if he's in pain?"

"That might be something you need to try."

"But the school is just going to call me to come pick him up!" I explode. Clearly, Dr. Lee doesn't have kids. "*You* are the abdominal doctor. Tell us what's going on!"

"Honey, I think Dr. Lee is trying—" my husband starts, but I cut him off.

"No. I want answers. And this doctor clearly can't provide them." I feel like Dr. Lee is dismissing not only me as the parent but also my child's pain. That's when I decide it's time for another doctor. "I want a second opinion. And," I add, pointing a finger at Dr. Lee, "I want to talk to *your* supervisor."

As the chairman of my department, I have been "the supervisor" that Mrs. Dennison demands to speak to on more than one occasion. In these situations, I have to stay balanced. Even if one of my physicians handled something differently from how I would have handled it, I need to help calm the situation while providing options for additional steps and maintaining the patient partnership. I simultaneously need to make it clear to the patient (and, as in Jonathan's case, the patient's family) that I am *listening to* them. I might acknowledge the situation like this: "From what you're sharing, it sounds like your son is really struggling, and it's having a significant impact on his schooling. That must be really challenging for you as a parent to witness and may even make you feel vulnerable or helpless. At this time, the challenge is finding a diagnosis for the symptoms." You don't want to take down another HCP, but you also don't want to enhance feelings of dismissal or make it seem as though medicine is the proverbial boys' club, with people just trying to protect one another.

When it comes to this balancing act, functional disorders can be particularly challenging. One of my attending physicians where I trained used to quote Carl Sagan, saying "absence of evidence is not evidence of absence." This is a truth that I frequently borrow in medical situations in which a functional disorder is suspected—there is no physiological basis for the patient's symptoms, but this does not diminish the patient's experience. And that's ultimately what this book is all about: the patient experience and how that is interpreted and communicated between the patient and the HCP.

Functional disorders are thought to make up as much as 20 percent of primary care consultations, with higher rates in specialties such as gastroenterology and neurology.[51] Risk factors for functional neurological symptoms include recent significant stress or trauma (emotional or physical); having an established neurological disorder, such as epilepsy;

and having a mental health condition, such as an anxiety disorder. Although the exact reasons for such disorders vary and aren't necessarily known, there is some support for the theory that functional neurological disorders may be related to dysfunctional emotional processing.[52] Depending on the situation, treatment for functional disorders can include behavioral therapy and cognitive behavioral therapy.

As a neurologist, I have seen functional disorders present as everything from Tourette's-like features to psychogenic non-epileptic seizures. In a non-epileptic seizure, a person presents with symptoms of what looks like seizure—but during the event, an EEG shows no electrical changes to indicate seizure. In Jonathan's case, there is no physical evidence of a physical GI issue being responsible for his stomach pains.

Communication Callout: Vulnerable Patients

In this chapter's opening anecdote, the patient is a child with unexplained stomach pains—sometimes an indicator of physical or emotional trauma or even of abuse or neglect. Members of the healthcare system have a duty to report suspected abuse or neglect to the appropriate authorities. In the case of vulnerable patients who cannot advocate for themselves, this need becomes even more pressing. There are 600,000 confirmed cases of child abuse yearly in the US, and for every incident of child abuse or neglect that's reported, it is estimated that there are two that go unreported.[53] When these concerns exist, they are complicated by a fear of being wrong—but patient safety is always the biggest concern. The **American Medical Association** provides a good review on how to handle these situations in the healthcare setting, which I've linked in Appendix B.

The approach to managing functional disorders has to be very cautious. If HCPs are not sensitive when delivering the diagnosis, the patient's or the family's perception may be that it is being suggested that the patient is "faking it," or that the symptoms are not real. The lived experience and the associated impairment are very real. The expected underlying pathophysiological cause is not. Consider how some bodies react to stress by showing physical symptoms, such as an upset stomach. In my case, I am now a confident public speaker, but I used to have an upset stomach for days before speaking events.

Functional disorders impact how the body's systems function but not as a result of change in body structure or any other measurable change. In the world of medicine, where we want concrete diagnoses, backed by tests, histories, and exams, this can be challenging for patients and HCPs alike. The question is, how do we avoid this turning into ill feelings that both sides take out on one another?

Service Recovery: Tapping into the EQ Superpower

When healing fractured relationships, that EQ we talked about in the book's early chapters becomes mission critical. In the case of a communication breakdown, the most important first step is usually to hit pause. For HCPs, take time to breathe before moving on to the next encounter, because you don't want to bring a defensive energy into the next interaction. This decompression is also important for minimizing burnout risk.

After a cooldown period, both sides need to exercise some self-awareness and ask themselves the following:

- What was my role in the communication breakdown?

- What words and actions did I use to convey my message?
- How was my message intended?
- How might my message have been received? Was it received as intended?
- Is anything influencing my communication negatively, such as implicit bias?
- Could there be a way to communicate my point more effectively; for example, with a visual instead of words?
- What is my end goal in this interaction?

When considering possible barriers standing in the way of communication, it can help to revisit the many factors that impact how messages are intended and received, as discussed in the first chapter. Here's a recap:

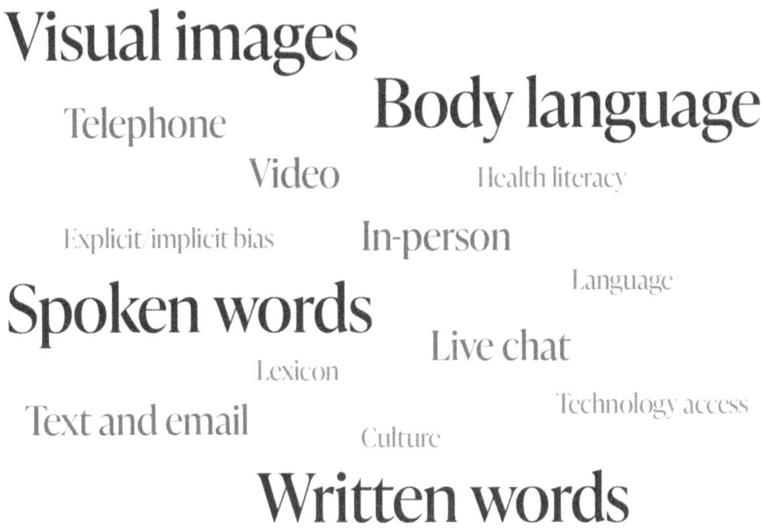

Figure 9.1: Factors that influence communication in healthcare and can impact breakdowns in understanding.

For patients, the issue in fractured relationships is often one of not feeling listened to. In this case, it's useful to turn to the progress map. What is the end goal of your wellness journey? Have you communicated this to the HCP and, if necessary, reiterated it? Having a physical copy of your symptom diary and progress map on hand, with your objectives clearly stated, helps everyone refocus and see the journey as it is experienced. For HCPs, the issue may simply be about validating the patient's concerns. At the same time, medical information still needs to be communicated clearly and objectively.

For both HCPs and patients, redirecting the conversation can help. This can mean using phrases such as the following:

- I am listening to what you're saying, but for the moment, I would like us to focus on XYZ first.
- I want to address that point shortly, but can we stay on XYZ right now?
- I understand your concern and will address it. However, I'd like to discuss XYZ first.

With that stated, sometimes the best thing to do is to pull in another person—to create balance, not to bully. Call on another expert. Pull in the supervisor. Send in the nurse that the patient or their family like. This gives both the HCP and the patient some distance without leaving the patient feeling deserted. Healthcare is a team effort, and a great, collaborative staff member is invaluable in diffusing a tense situation.

The importance of a team-based approach is also seen in second opinions. In the opening anecdote, Mrs. Dennison says she wants a second opinion. This is valid, and it's something I encourage patients and my team to advocate for, especially in cases in which there is a perception of unresolved concerns. The key here is to make sure the door remains open for communication and care. The HCP might even suggest a referral and add something to the effect of, "I always encourage a second opinion, especially when there are ongoing concerns that I have not been able to fully resolve. It introduces an opportunity to get another view with a fresh set of eyes. Please know that a second opinion does not cause obligation in any direction. If you wish to continue care there or return here, both are great options, and I support you either way."

There are also instances in which successful service recovery means terminating the relationship between the HCP and the patient. Not all relationships work, and you can't be everything to everyone. Having that self-recognition and social awareness is critically important to ensuring self-preservation and optimizing care. An HCP can tell a patient, "I am identifying that we are not able to make the best progress together, and I really want to make sure you get the right care. I think that what may end up being best is for me to introduce you to one of my colleagues, Dr. So-and-So, who is an expert in this area." It's not a question of "dumping" the patient but of using a team-based approach to align expectations and ensure positive outcomes.

Communication Callout: Service Recovery and Patients' Loved Ones

Fractured relationships in healthcare occur not only between the patient and the HCP. Often, there are fractures between patients and loved ones; for example, within families. There is a hint of this in the opening anecdote as the tension between Mr. and Mrs. Dennison becomes clear. Having a child with a chronic illness or special needs can place strain on a family. For example, parents of children with autism have a divorce rate of 80 percent.[54] Substance use disorders are another example of how illness can complicate relationships. Family and friends may distance themselves from individuals living with addiction because of problematic past behaviors and trust concerns.

HCPs may get caught in the middle of these strained relationships when addressing patients and their loved ones. This can contribute to an increased risk that service recovery will be needed because of misdirected emotions in an emotionally charged situation. Importantly, it is not the HCP's role to heal such rifts, but it is critical that they recognize them. The strained family relationship can impact the reporting of symptom burden or improvement, resulting in inconsistent information guiding diagnosis and treatment. Identifying and discussing concerns about how differing perspectives can impact care can be a step in the right direction. Broaching the topic is also a chance to point patients toward other resources, such as support groups.

Service recovery is an inevitable and essential part of healthcare delivery. It helps patients maintain a level of care that is optimal for them. It improves efficiency by helping to minimize patients ping-ponging around the system. In the big picture, service recovery can also help cut costs by making sure patients don't fall through the cracks and experience delayed care—problems that can result in their issues becoming more serious (and more costly to treat). From an ecosystem perspective, good service recovery keeps patients confident in the system—and, when patients leave satisfied, you are going to attract more patients. Finally, good service recovery reduces stress and tension for all involved. In short, it's in everyone's interests to learn how to put the wheels back on the bus when they're about to fall off.

A NARRATIVE CASE STUDY, REIMAGINED

When we left our opening anecdote, Mrs. Dennison was saying she wanted a second opinion and demanding to speak to Dr. Lee's supervisor. Let's see how Dr. Lee puts service recovery into action.

I take a breath and count to three in my head before replying to Mrs. Dennison, who is already on her feet, preparing to storm out. "Mrs. Dennison, I think it's a great idea to get a second opinion. I'm just as eager as you to make sure we get Jonathan feeling his best again."

"Oh." She blinks at me in surprise, taken aback, and plops back down in her seat.

"It's understandable to be upset when your child is having repeated symptoms of concern that are causing functional disruption to his daily life. The endoscopy and colonoscopy results rule out celiac and inflammatory bowel disease, which is good news. And all other prior testing has also been reassuring. With that said, there is no additional testing that would be appropriate at this time, and I suspect Jonathan has a functional abdominal disorder."

"A what?" The couple eyes me in confusion.

"This means that there is no physiological source of his symptoms. However, it doesn't mean that Jonathan's symptoms aren't real. Now we need to figure out how I can best help you moving forward. If that means referring you to another specialist, I'm happy to do so."

"But won't they just do the same test and find out the same thing?" Mr. Dennison cuts in. "I mean ... If the tests say he's fine ..." He drops his voice to a whisper as he says to his wife, "Maybe he's faking it? Maybe he just doesn't want to go to school."

"No!" Mrs. Dennison's voice is sharp. "He *cries*. He's not eating. He misses his friends at school. It's not that." She glares daggers at her husband.

I cut in quickly. "A functional disorder does not imply that he is faking it. In some situations, there can be associated features like school avoidance, either because of a fear of experiencing the symptoms in school or even a traumatic experience at school leading to functional symptoms. But in either case, it is not a purposeful act. This is a good place to be, as we've ruled out medical causes. However, Jonathan is still experiencing symptoms—behavior changes, lack of appetite, pain—and those are concerning."

"So, what do we do?" The Dennisons look to me.

***

I'm Jonathan's dad. I should protect him. But I feel totally helpless as we look to Dr. Lee. We need this doctor's help—and my wife is being so rude to him, I'm worried he's about to give us the boot. ***Can doctors fire patients?*** I wonder.

"A primary approach to treating functional disorders is cognitive behavioral therapy, or CBT, which is a form of psychology that can help modify Jonathan's recognition of symptoms and behaviors. We might also consider using medication to manage some of these issues, if needed," Dr. Lee says.

Is the doc saying Jonathan is crazy?! "Why would he need a psychologist?" I ask, suspicious.

"A psychologist trained in functional disorders can help Jonathan and the rest of us better understand the factors that contribute to his symptoms and what he can do to help redirect his response. This can decrease the frequency and severity of his symptoms. It is actually a treatment I recommend frequently to many patients with other neurological disorders. As they become empowered to recognize and respond to their bodies, overall outcomes may improve. As it stands now, the lack of predictability and the unknown are anxiety-provoking. In fact, this is probably causing anxiety for all of you."

I can't deny that.

"I'd suggest we start there," Dr. Lee continues. "In addition to a referral to a psychologist, I'd also like to refer Jonathan to a nutritionist. They can help ensure he is getting the nutrients he needs, even if he's eating less."

"It takes a village, huh, Doc?" I ask.

Dr. Lee nods. "I like to say it takes a team, as we are all shooting for the same goal. In this case, that goal is to help Jonathan feel good consistently and get back to school. I'd like to schedule a follow-up in four weeks. We want to keep tracking his weight and make sure the loss of appetite doesn't cause issues there."

"OK." I nod, relieved. My wife seems mollified, too. I'm glad we didn't storm out. We have a game plan, and that's at least one step forward. It feels as though we're getting a team of people behind us—and the follow-up is already set.

"It would also be helpful to me—and to any other physicians you might consult—if you all could start keeping a symptom diary for Jonathan. And I'd also like to create a progress map for him."

The doctor pulls out a couple of worksheet-like papers as he's talking: One is labeled ***Symptom Diary***, and the other is labeled ***Progress Map***. He explains how we can track things like Jonathan's pain, school days missed, and other symptoms—and how we can use the progress map to see how the changes we're implementing, like this CBT stuff, impact his symptoms.

"I think we can all agree on the end goal for Jonathan's journey," Dr. Lee goes on, pointing to the progress map. "We want Jonathan to be free of stomach pain so he can attend school regularly, play with his friends, and regain his appetite. Is that right?"

I nod, taking my wife's hand in mine. It feels like we're on the same page with the doctor. Looking at the progress map, I feel a tiny bit of hope.

Here, we see Dr. Lee validate the parents' concerns. Using tools we've discussed in this book, such as the symptom diary and the progress map, the doctor further makes it clear that he's not "giving up" on Jonathan's case. At the same time, Dr. Lee is providing the medical resources Jonathan needs, including a psychology referral. Mr. and Mrs. Dennison feel that they have been listened to and end up being amenable to working with Dr. Lee going forward. As Mr. Dennison himself recognizes, it now feels as though a team is behind them.

COMMUNITY SUPPORT

Rather than focusing on a disease-specific resource section, in this chapter, I want to take the opportunity to highlight ... the internet. Whether you are an HCP, a patient, a caregiver, a friend, or a family member, there is a treasure trove of resources online. Google can be your gateway to finding anything from support groups to clinical trials. Proceed with caution, recognizing what types of sites offer fact-based information versus which ones are clickbait. Academic sites (.edu), government sites (.gov), and sites affiliated with research and advocacy organizations, such as those listed in Appendix B, are good starting points. Should you take everything you read online as the gospel truth? Absolutely not! But the information you find there can be a valuable starting point to opening a discussion with the other members of the team in a wellness journey.

From the meet-and-greet to service recovery, we've looked at ways to enhance healthcare communication at every step. However, the world around us is evolving rapidly, not only in terms of healthcare delivery but also in terms of technology and how it shapes our social relationships. Old problems in communication are getting more complex as a result. One timely example is a study that looks at service recovery following medical AI service failure—the study's title asks, "Are you ready to forgive AI?"[55] Maybe some problems, such as service recovery, will get easier if we can lay the blame on robots, not people. The evolving tech presents many opportunities, both in the present—and for the future. What might that future look like?

> **Growth Opportunity: EQ Check-In**
>
> In service recovery, EQ becomes paramount—but it can be harder than ever to tap into our self-awareness and emotional regulation when we're feeling frustrated or defensive. How is your EQ? It's time to check in. Scan the QR code for a quick self-assessment.

Chapter 9 Endnotes

51 Ana Morelli, "Psychiatric Aspects of Chronic Physical Disease," *Medicine* 48, no. 12 (2020): 784–787, https://doi.org/10.1016/j.mpmed.2020.09.009, quoted in "Functional Disease," ScienceDirect, accessed December 4, 2024, https://www.sciencedirect.com/topics/medicine-and-dentistry/functional-disease.

52 Susannah Pick, Laura H. Goldstein, David L. Perez, and Timothy R. Nicholson, "Emotional Processing in Functional Neurological Disorder: A Review, Biopsychosocial Model and Research Agenda," *Journal of Neurology, Neurosurgery, and Psychiatry* 90, no. 6 (2019): 704–711, https://doi.org/10.1136/jnnp-2018-319201.

53 "National Statistics on Child Abuse," National Children's Alliance, accessed December 4, 2024, https://www.nationalchildrensalliance.org/media-room/old-national-statistics-on-child-abuse.

54 Ann Gold Buscho, "Divorce and Special Needs Children," *Psychology Today*, February 28, 2023, https://www.psychologytoday.com/intl/blog/a-better-divorce/202302/divorce-and-special-needs-children.

55 Aihui Chen, Yueming Pan, Longyu Li, and Yunshuang Yu, "Are You Willing to Forgive AI? Service Recovery from Medical AI Service Failure," *Industrial Management & Data Systems* 122, no. 11 (2022), https://doi.org/10.1108/IMDS-12-2021-0801.

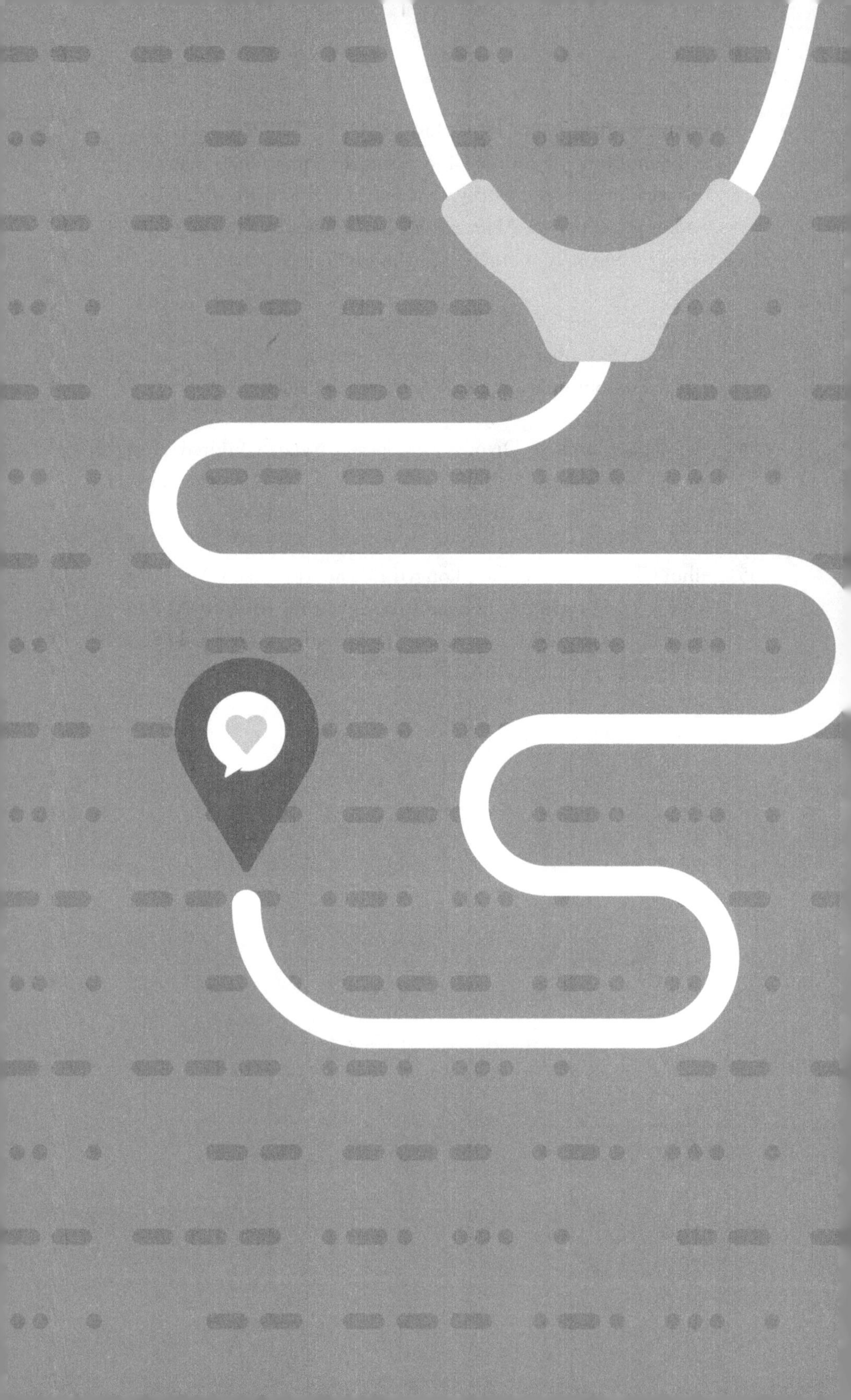

CHAPTER 10

Current Opportunities and Future Directions

The purpose of this chapter is to look at potential directions for the future of healthcare from a big-picture perspective, keeping in mind that there is always a context to consider. Every healthcare setting is unique and has different resources. Similarly, every individual's wellness journey is unique, including in terms of available opportunities.

NARRATIVE CASE STUDY: IMAGINING THE FUTURE

Imagine you wake up with a headache on a Sunday. Your primary care physician's offices are closed. Without getting out of bed, you reach for your phone and open the provider's app. You log into your account using biometric data—your fingerprint or face. Immediately, the AI-driven bot accesses your e-health record, which includes a full history of your past symptoms, diagnoses, and medical treatments.

How are you doing? the e-health chatbot asks you.

I've got a headache, you dictate to it.

I'm sorry to hear that! When did the headache start?

The chatbot takes you through questions about your headache, from when it began to how severe it is and whether you've taken any medications for it. It also asks other questions, including how much you slept the previous night, how much you drank, and whether you've eaten today.

At the end of the conversation, the chatbot tells you that it will record your notes in your personal symptom diary, which is a part of your permanent e-health record. It recommends a plan: *From your health record, I see that your only medication allergy is amoxicillin. Therefore, you can safely take ibuprofen. I suggest you take two 200 mg tablets of ibuprofen with one glass of water. Do you have ibuprofen, or should I put in a delivery order for the home address on file?*

You tell the chatbot you have ibuprofen at home—there's no need to have it sent over. Then you close the app, drag yourself out of bed, take your pills, and go back to sleep.

The next day, your primary care office contacts you via the same app: *We saw that you interacted with the chatbot. Did the medication help, or are you still experiencing symptoms?*

You tell them that you still have a headache and that you've now got a sore throat, too. They suggest making a telemedicine appointment that afternoon so an HCP can evaluate you. Based on that evaluation, they can decide on the next steps. At the beginning of the appointment, the doctor asks if he can use his AI scribe. Your conversation is transcribed into a note on the health app, and your symptom diary is updated automatically.

That afternoon, after a telemedicine appointment, your primary care physician recommends you come into the office in two days if your symptoms haven't improved. You get an appointment invite via the app, which is automatically added to your phone's calendar.

Two days later, you're in the office, seeing the physician in person. They have a full record of your last few days' symptoms, and you've already had an initial meet-and-greet over a telemedicine video call. Now they examine you in person, with a solid background established.

In this scenario, there is convenience, efficiency, and a continuous longitudinal model of care delivery with clear, ongoing, closed-loop communication. There is a first-line response through technology that gathers relevant information and provides immediate benefits while laying the foundation for subsequent support. A streamlined and cost-effective care pathway is created.

Ongoing development of remote patient monitoring (RPM) and diagnostics are continuing to expand possibilities and even reinvent what healthcare looks like. Say the patient reporting headaches also lives with hypertension, and their blood pressure is automatically recorded and reported to the app from home. The primary care physician could reach out proactively and say, "I see that you've been having increasing headaches. I also know that we've been having difficulty controlling your blood pressure. I'd like to make sure that those two things are not playing into one another, because the headache pain can make your blood pressure higher—and your blood pressure could be causing your pain." The physician could then send a twenty-four-hour blood pressure monitor to the patient that collects regular blood pressure readings and uploads them to a cloud storage system.

AI can comb through those readings constantly and raise a virtual red flag in case of concerning anomalies. With consistent use, it can even recognize patient-specific patterns.

Thanks to its learning capabilities and ability to rapidly sift through vast swaths of data, AI is already being used in areas of medicine such as radiology diagnostics. While some suggest that AI interferes with radiologists' performance,[56] others argue that it can improve accuracy and efficiency, allowing for more personalized healthcare delivery.[57] In short, the reviews are mixed, as people are still figuring out if, when, and how to best integrate such tools. However, one thing is certain: AI isn't going anywhere. By 2030, it's projected that healthcare industry spending on AI applications will exceed $200 *billion*.[58]

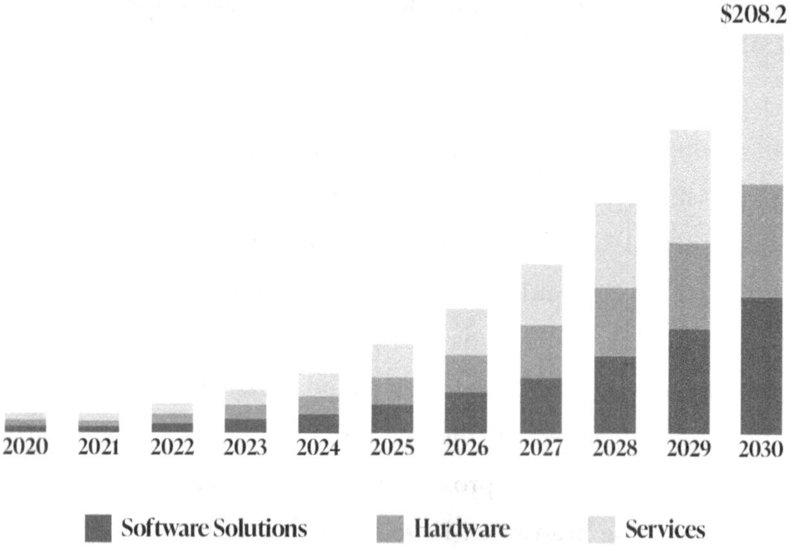

Figure 10.1: US AI in the healthcare market, size by component, 2020–2030 spending projections (USD). Amardeep Rawat, "Top Healthcare Trends That Will Redefine the Industry in 2025," Appinventiv, December 27, 2024, https://appinventiv.com/blog/healthcare-app-trends.

The bottom line is that tech holds amazing possibilities—if we harness it appropriately. And that's going to mean maintaining EQ, which underscores all effective healthcare communication.

Technology Is Part of the Solution, Not *THE* Solution

All of this might sound like something out of a sci-fi novel. But we aren't that far from it. For instance, the health system where I work has partnered with Best Buy Health to allow for hospital-level care and RPM at home. The Best Buy Geek Squad helps deliver and install the necessary equipment in the patient's home, while a healthcare team schedules appointments at the home—but mainly uses remote services for ongoing care. This can be a game-changer for patients in need of constant monitoring or care, especially if they face mobility challenges.

Such connected technologies aren't just great for gathering patient data; they're also valuable for the HCPs who need to share that data. One of the biggest challenges we see in healthcare right now is that there are a lot of point solutions without a lot of networking between them. You might have one device that measures heart rate, another that monitors sleep–wake cycles, and another that checks blood sugar. Compiling all that information in one spot requires an added step. As innovation explodes, we risk becoming overwhelmed with data if we don't find ways to qualify, synthesize, and streamline it.

This applies not only to medical data but also to administrative information. At the health system where I work, we frequently attempt to use an approach called the command center of care, where all information is centered in a single oversight system. We try to encourage patients to always enter the system through the "digital front door." This allows ease of access and consolidates the patient's record and resources immediately in one easy-access hub—health plans, insurance details, billing paperwork, test results, medical records. This information can be accessed by the healthcare team, improving efficiency. For example, when evaluating a patient for a specific therapy, the HCP can easily reference the patient's digital medical records to identify a treatment that's on formulary with their insurance.

These kinds of communication epicenters are likely going to become more prevalent in the future. They let us step back from a pigeonhole view of healthcare, allowing for holistic approaches that treat the patient as a whole human and not just as a single symptom or disease that needs attention at a single interaction.

With that stated, I won't pretend that it's going to be some perfect utopia. The proliferation of data presents concerns as well as opportunities. Beyond collecting data, what about analyzing it—what does it mean in real time, for the actual patient? When do we act on what the data is telling us? And then there are the legalities, such as who controls the data and how it might be stored safely. What if there is a dysfunction in a device or in the transmission of the data collected? As healthcare becomes more digitized, legal and operational concerns arise.

There are also cost issues to consider. For example, insurance currently only covers the use of one RPM device per patient, per month. The cardiologist may want to prioritize an at-home RPM that has a specific algorithm for heart-rate monitoring, while the pulmonologist may prefer an alternative device relevant to their department. You can only bill for one per month; someone isn't going to get paid. Plus, there is the added cost to patient quality of life. How many devices does one need to wear, and how many times? The ability to use a singular device can improve patient comfort and convenience—and likely costs as well.

Inevitably, there are going to be gaps in access to such modern care. Internet access can vary. Technology access can vary. The scenario described in this chapter's futuristic opening anecdote—is that going to be available to everyone, everywhere? This kind of modern concierge care would ideally help remove disparities in healthcare systems. However, there is a chance that it could widen the gap.

Overall, I think technology can help us in a lot of ways. By taking care of more tedious tasks, such as data collection, tech can free up our energy to focus on the one thing the tech can't replace—the human aspect. And we will need to fall back on that humanity to guide the implementation of technology ethically. How do we train AI to avoid bias, for instance? These are questions not only for HCPs but also for IT professionals, lawyers, ethicists, health systems, politicians, lobbyists, the FDA … A lot of people are shaping this future.

Communication Still Starts with EQ

Yes, when we hide behind screens, technology can hinder communication. But it can also improve communication! With tech, we have the possibility of putting the person back at the center. The bots, the diagnostic tools, the AI—all of this helps to gather, centralize, and organize information. And information—about the patient, their condition, their history—is what we need to develop personalized treatment plans. When HCPs have admin and time-consuming tasks (such as writing notes) taken off their plate, they gain valuable time, which can go toward professional self-investment, further augmenting their EQ and enhancing communication.

However, as always, it's not just on the HCP's shoulders. Good communication still requires shared accountability, and tech won't change that. For example, the most cutting-edge, at-home monitoring device won't do any good if the patient doesn't implement it as directed. And that accountability goes beyond patients and providers.

Health systems, insurers, advocacy groups, families and friends, the extended community—all are relevant in the patient's journey now, and they will continue to be. Technology can simply make the journey easier. If patients have been driving a beat-up old Volvo, tech can make it feel as though they're cruising to their wellness objectives in a shiny new Porsche.

Either way, patients still need their trusted GPS to guide them toward their desired destination. And to make the most of that GPS, patients need to know what information to give it. Toward that end, tools such as a symptom diary and a progress map can be helpful. Simple as they may seem, both are valuable for conveying essential information. And when communication improves, both sides benefit. Less stress for HCPs. Better outcomes for patients. Improved understanding for all.

When our message is perceived and received as we intend it, productive and positive relationships flourish. In medicine, this allows for those principles I'm always hammering home (my medical residents can attest) to be put into practice again and again. I leave you with them now: trust, respect, communication, best-in-class care, and teamwork!

Resource Wrap-Up

Throughout the book, I've shared various resources that HCPs and patients alike can use to enhance healthcare communication. Links to these resources can be found in Appendix B. You can also visit my website for more—just scan the QR code.

Chapter 10 Endnotes

56 Ekaterina Pesheva, "Does AI Help or Hurt Human Radiologists' Performance? It Depends on the Doctor," Harvard Medical School, March 2024, https://hms.harvard.edu/news/does-ai-help-or-hurt-human-radiologists-performance-depends-doctor.

57 Mohamed Khalifa and Mona Albadawy, "AI in Diagnostic Imaging: Revolutionising Accuracy and Efficiency," *Computer Methods and Programs in Biomedicine Update* 5 (2024): 100146, https://doi.org/10.1016/j.cmpbup.2024.100146.

58 Amardeep Rawat, "Top Healthcare Trends That Will Redefine the Industry in 2025," Appinventiv, December 27, 2024, https://appinventiv.com/blog/healthcare-app-trends.

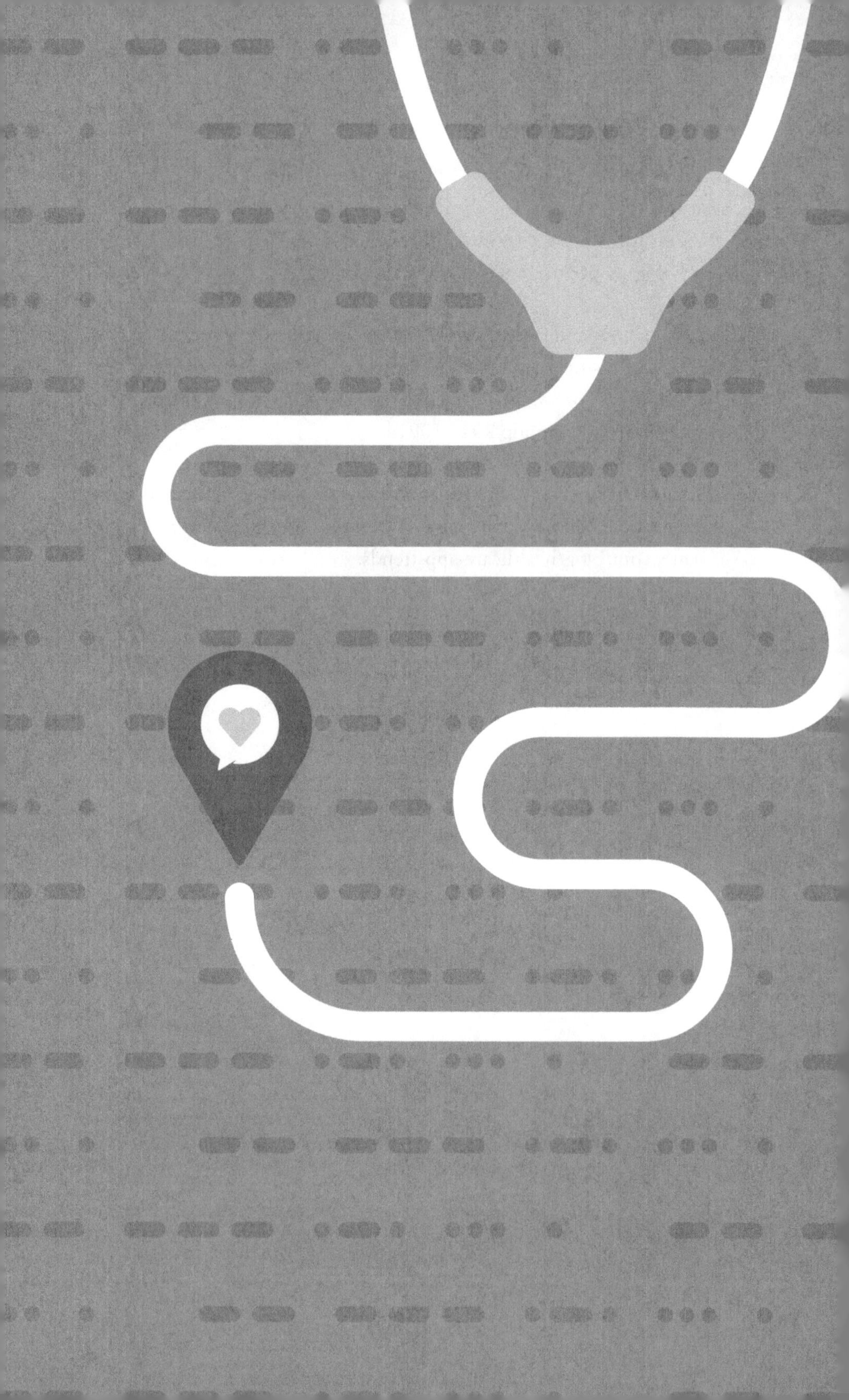

CONCLUSION

Set Your Intention

My personal intention with this book is a call to action. Whoever you are, be it a patient, an HCP, a caregiver, a nurse, an administrator … don't wait for the future. The future is now. Through this book, I hope you've developed some greater awareness of EQ and considered how to fine-tune your own self-awareness and self-management. Maybe you have seen yourself or someone you know in some of the fictional anecdotes—and perhaps this has allowed you to identify ways in which you can communicate with greater intention and awareness.

Looking back on my own experience with my mom, I'm grateful that I have learned how to be a partner to her on her healthcare journey, through all its phases. Years ago, this meant helping her reenter the healthcare system after being "lost to follow-up" in the wake of her MS diagnosis. Over the past year, being a partner to her in her healthcare journey has meant helping her navigate a cancer diagnosis. As the only doctor in the family, my responsibility was to ensure that accurate information was being communicated between my mom's HCPs and our family. It took all of us as a team—me, my dad, my siblings, my extended family—to navigate the journey.

Over my career, I've gotten all kinds of feedback—the good, the bad, and the ugly! It's not always easy to receive—such as this book's opening comment from a patient's sister: "During our first conversation, all I could think about was how much I hated you." However, the negatives have helped me grow.

More recently, a respected colleague gave me some positive feedback, telling me, "I am always impressed by how you speak to patients and their families. That is a big part of what makes you such an excellent clinician, and it is very important that your trainees learn that aspect of medicine from you." With this book, I hope I can reach beyond the immediate sphere of my trainees and help others learn how to advocate for themselves and for those around them.

I can't change healthcare alone. But I will continue to be a relentless advocate for a better way to experience healthcare. Hopefully, you now also desire a model of healthcare that is represented by a continuous, longitudinal, patient-directed partnership.

Words matter. Make yours count.

APPENDIX A

Glossary

Accountability: A commitment to performing the roles and responsibilities of a member of the team, fostering trust and respect, with the goal of supporting individuals in achieving optimal patient-desired outcomes.

AIDET™: A model for patient communication built on the following steps: **A**cknowledge, **I**ntroduce, **D**uration, identify next steps, **E**xplanation, **T**hank you.

Chief complaint (CC): The reason a person is presenting for care.

C-I-CARE: A model for patient communication built on the framework of **C**onnecting with people by calling them by their proper names; **I**ntroducing yourself; **C**ommunicating what you're going to do and why; **A**sking permission before every action; **R**esponding to patient questions or requests promptly; and **E**xiting courteously and always with an explanation of what will come next.

Communication: The process of generating meaning by sending and receiving symbolic cues that are influenced by multiple contexts.

Emotional quotient (EQ): The ability to perceive, use, understand, manage, and handle emotions. Sometimes referred to as emotional intelligence, or EI.

Empathy: The ability to understand and share the feelings of another.

Guiding Partner Specialist (GPS): An HCP who guides the patient's journey. The patient inputs their desired destination into the GPS (say, a life free of XYZ symptoms), and the GPS should be able to tell them the possible routes to get there, how long it may take, detours that might occur, and when they need to completely reroute.

Healthcare partner (HCP): A healthcare partner may be a doctor, a nurse, a physical therapist, a psychiatrist, a psychologist, a pharmacist—any healthcare professional who plays a role in the patient's care journey.

History of presenting illness (HPI): A chronological description of the development of the patient's present illness from the first sign and/or symptom or from the previous encounter to the present.

Illness script: An organized mental summary of an HCP's knowledge of a disease. Classically, the components of an illness script fall into three categories—predisposing conditions, pathophysiological insult, and clinical consequences.

Patient-valued care: A healthcare model that measures the value of care according to how much value is provided to the patient, as defined by the patient.

Patient-valued outcomes: Healthcare outcomes that are defined and prioritized by the patient. Such outcomes might include eliminating a certain symptom or resuming an activity that was previously impossible for health reasons. There is no set quantitative metric; the patient determines the metric to be used.

Point solution: Individual services designed to provide health-, wellness-, and/or condition-based services in the healthcare ecosystem.

Value-based care: A healthcare model that exclusively holds providers accountable for improving patient outcomes by measuring the quality of healthcare and patient outcomes in relation to the cost of care.

Value-based outcomes: Providers are paid based on patient health outcomes; the "value" of value-based outcomes, as typically understood, is purely fiscal.

Paternalistic model of care: In a healthcare context, a care-delivery model in which an HCP makes decisions for a patient.

Self-awareness: Exercising awareness of one's own feelings, motives, and desires.

Self-management: Exercising control over how one responds to influences, both internal and external.

Shared care model of care delivery: In a healthcare context, a care delivery model in which HCPs and patients work together to determine the course of care.

Social awareness: The ability to differentiate between intentional and unintentional communication, empathizing and considering alternative perspectives, especially those of people of different backgrounds and cultures.

Social management: A person's ability to act in a socially aware way, considering alternative perspectives, especially those of people with different backgrounds and cultures.

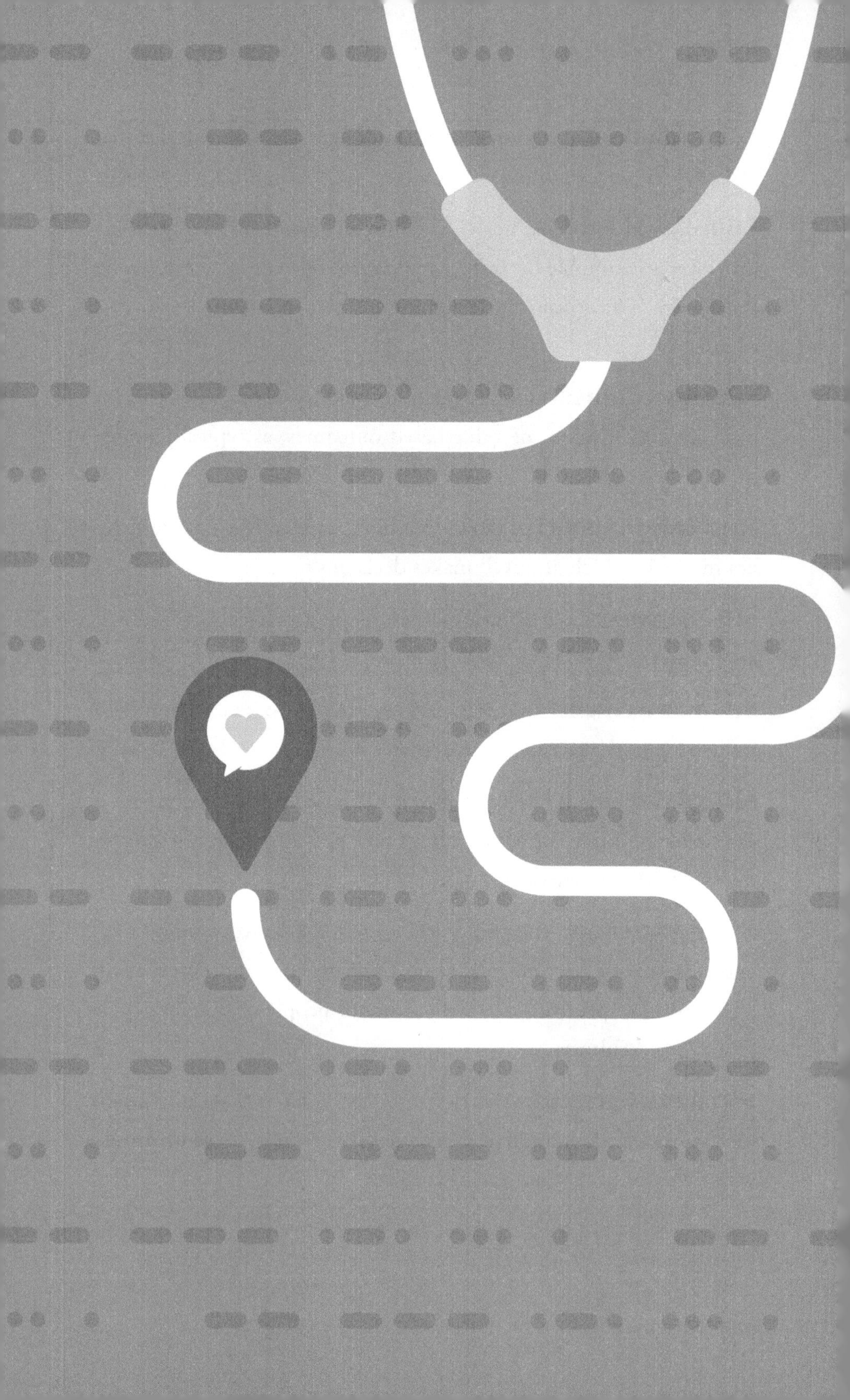

APPENDIX B

Resources

Resources are listed in the order in which they are mentioned in the book.

Wake Up Narcolepsy

- Event calendar of virtual and in-person events across all ages.
    - https://www.wakeupnarcolepsy.org/events/month/
- Free online support groups for individuals with narcolepsy and their families.
    - https://www.wakeupnarcolepsy.org/community/
- Patient, family, and caregiver education resources.
    - https://www.wakeupnarcolepsy.org/about/what-is-narcolepsy/
- Clinical trials and research updates for HCPs.
    - https://www.wakeupnarcolepsy.org/research/
- Grants and funding for researchers.
    - https://www.wakeupnarcolepsy.org/research/grants/

DAMM Good Sleep

- Various sleep health resources.
    - https://www.dammgoodsleep.com/

American Cancer Society

- 24/7 support line in more than two hundred languages for those who are facing a cancer diagnosis or know someone facing a diagnosis.
    - https://www.fightcancer.org/american-cancer-society-resources-cancer-patients/

National Cancer Institute

- Educational information about different types of cancers, diagnosis and staging, and clinical trials.
    - https://www.cancer.gov/

National Comprehensive Cancer Network

- Resources for physicians as well as patients and caregivers.
    - https://www.nccn.org/

Centers for Disease Control and Prevention

- Information about obesity.
    - https://www.cdc.gov/obesity/index.html

American Society for Nutrition

- Dietary resources relating to obesity.
    - https://nutrition.org/obesity-resources/

Obesity Action Coalition

- Evidence-based education about obesity.
    - https://www.obesityaction.org/

American Migraine Foundation

- The latest in migraine research.
    - https://americanmigrainefoundation.org/

American Headache Society

- Information on the study and treatment of headaches and face pain. Physician members can attend upcoming events, access research grants, and more.
    - https://americanheadachesociety.org/

Autism Speaks

- Materials to support people with autism in different life stages, from pediatric to adult.
    - https://www.autismspeaks.org/

Autism Society

- Advocacy and educational materials, including information about autism screening.
    - https://autismsociety.org/

Simons Foundation Autism Research Initiative Foundation

- Autism-related funding and research initiatives.
    - https://www.sfari.org/

Colin Farrell Foundation

- Resources to help adults with intellectual disability live successfully.
    - https://colinfarrellfoundation.org/

Allergy and Asthma Network

- A great starting point for patients seeking information.
    - https://allergyasthmanetwork.org/

Asthma and Allergy Foundation of America

- Asthma action plan template to help patients stay on top of care.
    - https://aafa.org/asthma/asthma-treatment/asthma-treatment-action-plan/

Respiratory Health Association

- Videos that cover everything from asthma warning signs to allergens and irritants that can trigger asthma.
    - https://resphealth.org/healthy-lungs/asthma/living-with-asthma/

National Organization for Rare Disorders

- A centralized resource that represents all rare disease resources for patients, HCPs, researchers, and advocates.
    - https://rarediseases.org/

Penn Medicine: University of Pennsylvania Health System

- A primer on how religious beliefs impact patient beliefs.
    - https://www.uphs.upenn.edu/pastoral/resed/diversity_points.html

American Academy of Sleep Medicine

- Resources to improve knowledge and awareness of sleep disorders, including tips for finding a credentialed specialist and how to become involved in sleep advocacy.
    - https://sleepeducation.org/

American Medical Association

- Review and information on how to handle suspected abuse or neglect in a healthcare setting.
    - https://www.ama-assn.org/delivering-care/physician-patient-relationship/you-suspect-patient-being-abused-what-should-you-do

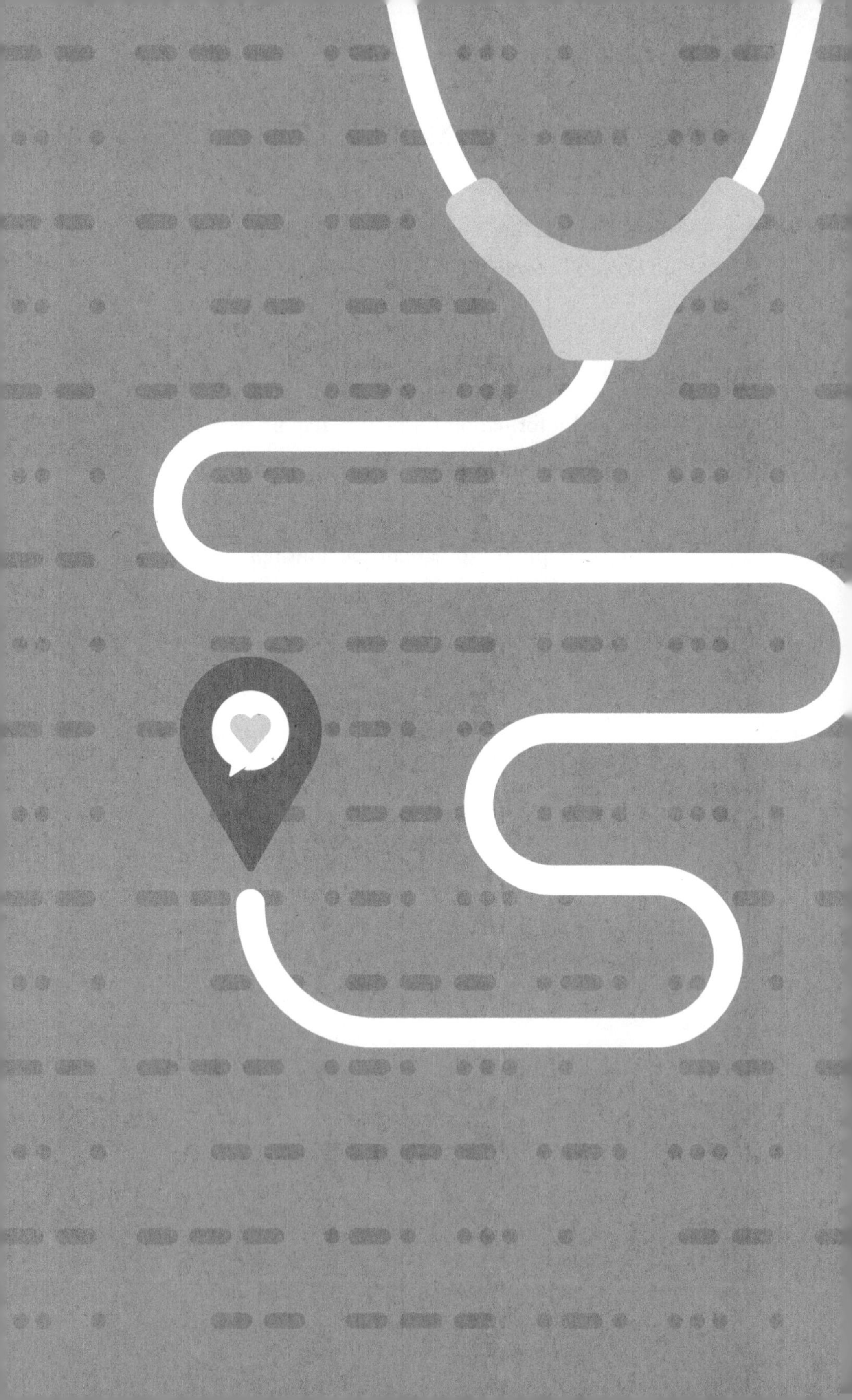

ACKNOWLEDGMENTS

A specific expression of acknowledgment and gratitude to Wake Up Narcolepsy (WUN), a national nonprofit that has been empowering individuals and communities since 2008. They exist to drive awareness and education with goals that include reducing time between symptom onset and diagnosis and ensuring improved, accessible treatments. WUN offers several unique virtual support groups and in-person events and has contributed millions toward clinical research in the narcolepsy space.

Thank you for the honor of being recognized with the inaugural award as the Physician Champion for Patient Advocacy and for your support in helping make this book a reality. Thank you also for the resources you provide for countless people on their medical journeys and for serving as an educational resource across the healthcare ecosystem.

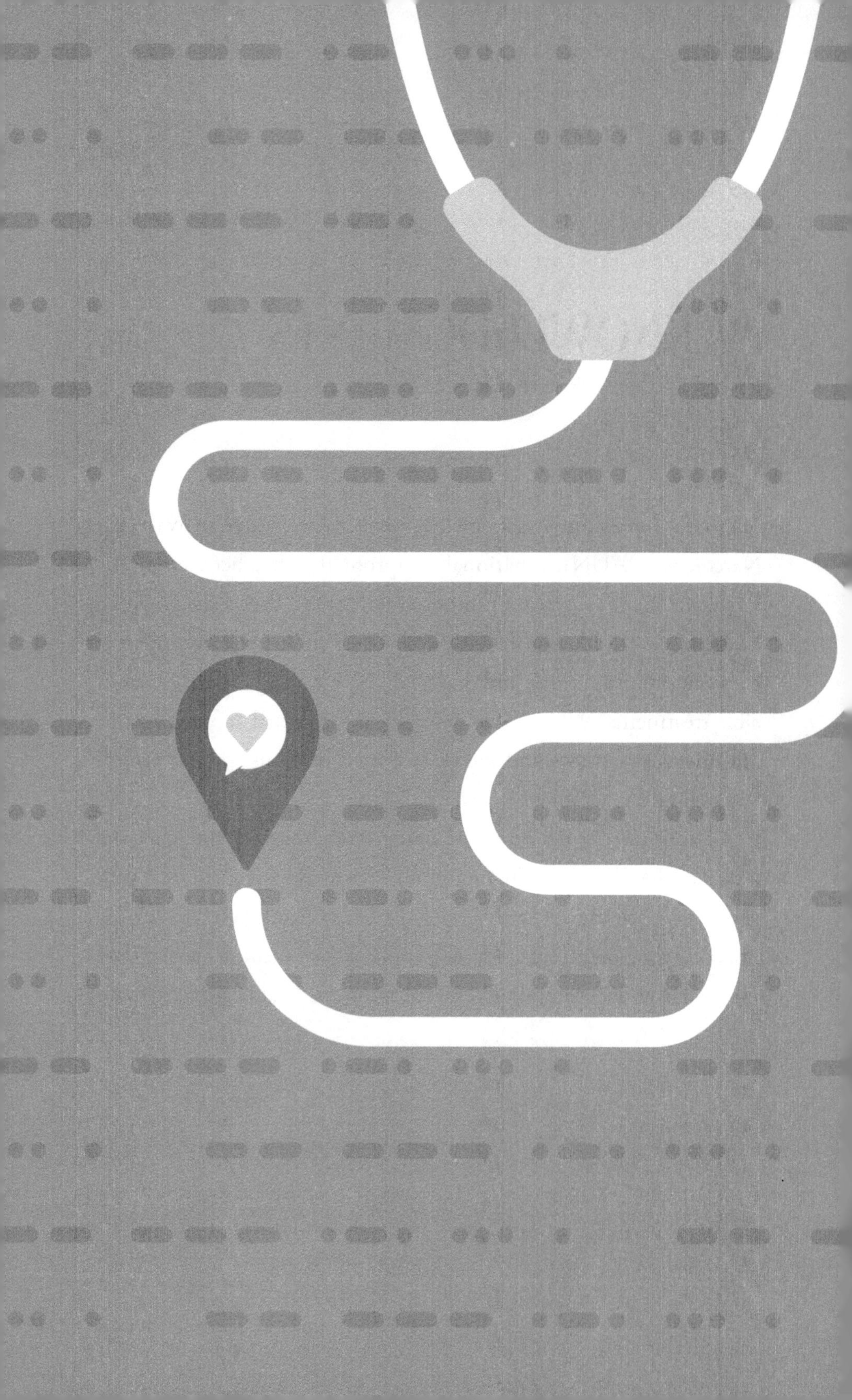

ABOUT THE AUTHOR

Dr. Anne Marie Morse is a board-certified adult neurologist with special qualifications in child neurology, as well as a fellowship-trained and board-certified sleep medicine specialist. She is the Division Chief of Child Neurology and Pediatric Sleep Medicine at Janet Weis Children's Hospital, Geisinger (Danville, Pennsylvania). Despite her pediatric titles, Dr. Morse's clinical practice, research, educational efforts, community outreach, advisory positions, and advocacy reach across all ages. She is an internationally recognized key opinion leader; a distinguished educator; a Press Ganey–recognized national top 10 percent clinician for exceptional patient experience; an Alpha Omega Alpha honor society member; and one of modern healthcare's recognized "top 40 under 40."

Dr. Morse has proudly embraced her reputation as a healthcare disruptor, recognizing the need to move away from the current model of siloed episodic transactional care to a patient-directed longitudinal model of continuous care. She is a staunch advocate for emboldening the patient voice and creating a healthcare dynamic in which medical professionals can collaborate in care delivery as healthcare partners (HCPs) with patients in their care journey and in which both HCPs and patients are able to rely on the broader healthcare ecosystem to seamlessly meet all needs along the wellness journey. To facilitate the change needed to achieve patient-desired outcomes and improved economic stewardship in healthcare, Dr. Morse focuses on all the tools available to improve communication across the healthcare ecosystem and within the community.

Leaning into EQ skill-building and taking a systems-based approach, a full ecosystem includes, prioritizes, and elevates patient and community voice and needs; acknowledges the escalating rates of burnout and cynicism in healthcare; attempts to better navigate the increasing complexity of medicine; and offers a financially feasible effort to achieve the outcomes that all involved parties value.

As a healthcare leader, educator, advocate, and innovator, Dr. Morse relies on five basic principles to be successful:

- Trust
- Respect
- Communication
- Best-in-class practice
- Teamwork

The keystone of this pentad is effective communication. To develop and maintain a thriving partnership that results in a personalized wellness journey and enables the ability to provide the right care to the right person at the right time, a fully transparent expression of status, needs, progress, and goals is necessary.

ENDNOTES

1 Erin C. Golden, MD, and Melissa C. Lipford, MD, "Narcolepsy: Diagnosis and Management," *Cleveland Clinic Journal of Medicine* 85, no. 12 (2018): 959–969, https://doi.org/10.3949/ccjm.85a.17086.

2 Kate E. Humphrey, Melissa Sundberg, Carly E. Milliren, Dionne A. Graham, and Christopher P. Landrigan, "Frequency and Nature of Communication and Handoff Failures in Medical Malpractice Claims," *Journal of Patient Safety* 18, no. 2 (2022): 130–137, https://doi.org/10.1097/PTS.0000000000000937.

3 Richard R. Hurtig, Rebecca M. Alper, and Benjamin Berkowitz, "The Cost of Not Addressing the Communication Barriers Faced by Hospitalized Patients," *Perspectives of the ASHA Special Interest Groups* 12, no. 3 (2018): 99–112, https://doi.org/10.1044/persp3.SIG12.99.

4 "Amazon Takes Another Shot at Health Care, This One a Virtual Care Service That Costs $9 Per Month," The Associated Press, November 9, 2023, https://apnews.com/article/amazon-medical-membership-b961a006c24f82a839f971708b609800.

5 Angelina Jolie, "My Medical Choice," *The New York Times*, May 14, 2013, https://www.nytimes.com/2013/05/14/opinion/my-medical-choice.html.

6 Jens B. Stephansen, Alexander N. Olesen, Mads Olsen, Aditya Ambati, Eileen B. Leary, Hyatt E. Moore et al., "Neural Network Analysis of Sleep Stages Enables Efficient Diagnosis of Narcolepsy," *Nature Communications* 9, no. 5229 (2018), https://doi.org/10.1038/s41467-018-07229-3.

7 Victoria Leonard, "Types of Communication" in *COMS 246: Interpersonal* Communication, course materials (College of the Canyons), accessed December 4, 2024, https://socialsci.libretexts.org/Courses/College_of_the_Canyons/COMS_246%3A_Interpersonal_Communication_(Leonard)/1%3A_Introduction_to_Communication/1.1%3A_Types_of_Communication.

8 Ibid.

9 John W. Ayers, Adam Poliak, Mark Dredze, Eric C. Leas, Zechariah Zhu, Jessica B. Kelley et al., "Comparing Physician and Artificial Intelligence Chatbot Responses to Patient Questions Posted to a Public Social Media Forum," *JAMA Internal Medicine* 183, no. 6 (April 2023): 589-–596, https://doi.org/10.1001/jamainternmed.2023.1838.

10 Jun Watanabe, Hiroyuki Teraura, Akihisa Nakamura, and Kazuhiko Kotani, "Telemental Health in Rural Areas: A Systematic Review," *Journal of Rural Medicine* 18, no. 2 (April 2023): 50–54, https://doi.org/10.2185/jrm.2022-059.

11 Carly McCord, Fred Ullrich, Kimberly A. S. Merchant, Divya Bhagianadh, Knute D. Carter, EveLynn Nelson et al., "Comparison of In-Person vs. Telebehavioral Health Outcomes from Rural Populations Across America," *BMC Psychiatry* 22, no. 778 (2022), https://doi.org/10.1186/s12888-022-04421-0.

12 Marshall, Angela. *Dismissed: Tackling the Biases that Undermine Our Health Care*. S.l.: CITADEL PR, 2024.

13 "What Is Value-Based Healthcare?" *NEJM Catalyst*, January 1, 2017, https://catalyst.nejm.org/doi/full/10.1056/CAT.17.0558.

14 Oliver J. Canfell, Leanna Woods, Yasaman Meshkat, Jenna Krivit, Brinda Gunashanhar, Christine Slade et al., "The Impact of Digital Hospitals on Patient and Clinician Experience: Systematic Review and Qualitative Evidence Synthesis," *Journal of Medical Internet Research* 26 (March 2024): e47715, https://doi.org/10.2196/47715.

15 J. D. Mayer, P. Salovey, D. R. Caruso, and G. Sitarenios, "Emotional Intelligence as a Standard Intelligence," *Emotion* 1, no. 3 (2001): 232–242, https://doi.org/10.1037/1528-3542.1.3.232.

16 Richard E. Boyatzis, Daniel Goleman, and Kenneth Rhee, "Clustering Competence in Emotional Intelligence: Insights from the Emotional Competence Inventory," in *The Handbook of Emotional Intelligence: Theory, Development, Assessment, and Application at Home, School, and in the Workplace*, eds. R. Bar-On and J. D. A. Parker (Jossey-Bass/Wiley, 2000).

17 Nikhilesh Singh, Sweta Kulkarni, and Richa Gupta, "Is Emotional Intelligence Related to Objective Parameters of Academic Performance in Medical, Dental, and Nursing Students: A Systematic Review," *Education for Health (Abdingdon)* 33, no. 1 (2020): 8–12, https://doi.org/10.4103/efh.EfH_208_17.

18 John C. Licciardone, Yen Tran, Khang Ngo, David Toledo, Navya Peddireddy, and Subhash Aryal, "Physician Empathy and Chronic Pain Outcomes," *JAMA Network Open* 7, no. 4 (2024): e246026, https://doi.org/10.1001/jamanetworkopen.2024.6026.

19 Shama Kadadi and Shankargouda R. Bharamanaikar, "Role of Emotional Intelligence in Healthcare Industry," *Drishtikon: A Management Journal* 11, no. 1 (October 2020): 37, https://www.researchgate.net/publication/344955693_Role_of_Emotional_Intelligence_in_Healthcare_Industry.

20 Cy Wakeman, "Redefining Accountability in the Workplace," *Medium*, March 26, 2017, https://medium.com/@CyWakeman/redefining-accountability-in-the-workplace-1e880b4246d6.

21 Beth A. Lown, Julie Rosen, and John Marttila, "An Agenda for Improving Compassionate Care: A Survey Shows About Half of Patients Say Such Care is Missing," *Health Affairs (Millwood)* 30, no. 9 (2011): 1772–8, https://doi.org/10.1377/hlthaff.2011.0539.

22 Stephen R. Covey, *The 7 Habits of Highly Effective People: Powerful Lessons in Personal Change*, anniversary edition (Simon & Schuster, 2013).

23 Andriana M. Foiles Sifuentes, Monica Robledo Cornejo, Nien Chen Li, Maira A. Castaneda-Avila, Jennifer Tjia, and Kate L. Lapane, "The Role of Limited English Proficiency and Access to Health Insurance and Health Care in the Affordable Care Act Era," *Health Equity* 4, no. 1 (2020): 509–517, https://doi.org/10.1089/heq.2020.0057.

24 Mamata Pandey, R. Geoffrey Maina, Jonathan Amoyaw, Yiyan Li, Rejina Kamrul, C. Rocha Michaels et al., "Impacts of English Language Proficiency on Healthcare Access, Use, and Outcomes Among Immigrants: A Qualitative Study," *BMC Health Services Research* 21, no. 741 (2021): 1–13, https://doi.org/10.1186/s12913-021-06750-4.

25 Chandrika Divi, Richard G. Koss, Stephen P. Schmaltz, and Jerod M. Loeb, "Language Proficiency and Adverse Events in US Hospitals: A Pilot Study," *Journal of the International Society for Quality in Health Care* 19, no. 2 (2007): 60–67, https://doi.org/10.1093/intqhc/mzl069.

26 "Taking the Pulse on Physicians to Spur Action," The Physicians Foundation, accessed December 4, 2024, https://physiciansfoundation.org/surveys/.

27 Caroline E. Rassbach, Alyssa L. Bogetz, Nicola Orlov, Alisa McQueen, Vasudah Bhavaraju, David Mahoney et al., "The Effect of Faculty Coaching on Resident Attitudes, Confidence, and Patient-Rated Communication: A Multi-Institutional Randomized Controlled Trial," *Academic Pediatrics* 19, no. 2 (2018): 186–194, https://doi.org/10.1016/j.acap.2018.10.004.

28 Noam N. Levey, "In America, Cancer Patients Endure Debt on Top of Disease," *KFF Health News*, July 9, 2022, https://kffhealthnews.org/news/article/in-america-cancer-patients-endure-debt-on-top-of-disease/.

29 Thien T. Nguyen, "The Effect of AIDET Communications Delivered by Front Desk Staff on Patient Experience and Satisfaction at a Medical Practice" (doctorate thesis, Capella University, 2019), ProQuest Dissertations & Theses (13427293), https://www.proquest.com/openview/c584ec9cbf93119b13f345931407bafb.

30 Kun Fu, Shuping Li, and Sufen Lu, "Application and Effect Evaluation on Acknowledge-Introduce-Duration-Explanation-Thank You (AIDET) Communication Mode in Cataract Daytime Operation Nursing," *Annals of Eye Science* 5 (June 2020), https://doi.org/10.21037/aes.2020.03.01.

31 Tiffany Nguyen, "Implementing AIDET and Commit to Sit to Increase Patient Satisfaction in the Pediatric Outpatient Setting" (master's thesis, University of San Francisco, 2022), University of San Francisco Master's Projects and Capstones (1365), https://repository.usfca.edu/capstone/1365.

32 Andrea Mechanick Braverman, Elisabeth J. Kunkel, Leo Katz, Austin Katona, Theresa Heavens, Andrew Miller et al., "Do I Buy It? How AIDET™ Training Changes Residents' Values About Patient Care," *Journal of Patient Experience* 2, no. 1 (2015): 13–20, https://doi.org/10.1177/237437431500200104.

33 Sun-Ju She and Ying-Ying Xu, "Effect of CICARE Communication Nursing Model Combined with Motivational Psychological Intervention in Patients with Post-Intensive Care Unit Syndrome," *World Journal of Psychiatry* 13, no. 9 (2019): 707–713, https://doi.org/10.5498/wjp.v13.i9.707.

34 "Overweight & Obesity Statistics," National Institute of Diabetes and Digestive and Kidney Diseases, accessed December 4, 2024,

https://www.niddk.nih.gov/health-information/health-statistics/overweight-obesity.

35 M. van Berge Henegouwen, H. van Driel, and D. Kasteleijn-nolst trenité, "A Patient Diary as a Tool to Improve Medicine Compliance," *Pharmacy World and Science* 21 (1999): 21–24, https://doi.org/10.1023/A:1008627824731.

36 Bryan Hodge, "The Use of Symptom Diaries in Outpatient Care," *Family Practice* 20, no. 3 (2013): 24–28, https://www.aafp.org/pubs/fpm/issues/2013/0500/p24.html.

37 Michael A. Fischer, John B. McKinlay, Jeffrey N. Katz, Eric Gerstenberger, Felicia Trachtenberg, Lisa D. Marceau et al., "Physician Assessments of Drug Seeking Behavior: A Mixed Methods Study," *PLoS One* 12, no. 6 (2023): e0178690, https://doi.org/10.1371/journal.pone.0178690.

38 George Lindbeck, Manish I. Shah, Sabina Braithwaite, Jonathan R. Powell, Ashish R. Panchal, Lorin R. Brown et al., "Evidence-Based Guidelines for Prehospital Pain Management: Recommendations," *Prehospital Emergency Care* 27, no. 2 (2025): 144–153, https//doi.org/10.1080/10903127.2021.2018073; Saïd Hachimi-Idrissi, Viliam Dobias, Wolf E. Hautz, Robert Leach, Thomas C. Sauter, Idanna Sforzi et al., "Approaching Acute Pain in Emergency Settings; European Society for Emergency Medicine (EUSEM) Guidelines—Part 2: Management and Recommendations," *Internal Emergency Medicine* 15, no. 7 (2020): 1141–1155, https://doi.org/10.1007/s11739-020-02411-2.

39 Torie Grant, Emily Croce, and Elizabeth C. Matsui, "Asthma and the Social Determinants of Health," *CME Review* 128, no. 1 (2022): 5–11, https://doi.org/10.1016/j.anai.2021.10.002.

40 Tom Neltner and Kathy Seikel, "Pests Persist in Federally Subsidized Housing," National Center for Healthy Housing and US Environmental Protection Agency, accessed December 4, 2024, https://nchh.org/resource-library/Case_Study_Conditions_10-14-07.pdf.

41 Jamie Ducharme and Elijah Wolfson, "Your Zip Code Might Determine How Long You Live—and the Difference Could Be Decades," *Time*, June 17, 2019, https://time.com/5608268/zip-code-health/.

42 G. M. Murtagh, L. Furber, and A. L. Thomas, "Patient-Initiated Questions: How Can Doctors Encourage Them and Improve the Consultation Process? A Qualitative Study," *BMJ Open* 3, no. 10 (2013): e003112, https://doi.org/10.1136/bmjopen-2013-003112.

43 Joanna Burzyńska, Anna Bartosiewicz, and Paweł Januszewicz, "Dr. Google: Physicians—the Web—Patients Triangle: Digital Skills and Attitudes Towards e-Health Solutions Among Physicians in South Eastern Poland—a Cross-Sectional Study in a Pre-COVID-19 Era," *International Journal of Environmental Research and Public Health* 20, no. 2 (2023): 978, https://doi.org/10.3390/ijerph20020978.

44 "What is Asthma?" Allergy & Asthma Network, accessed December 4, 2024, https://allergyasthmanetwork.org/what-is-asthma/.

45 "Rare Disease Day: Frequently Asked Questions," National Organization for Rare Disorders, accessed December 4, 2024, https://rarediseases.org/wp-content/uploads/2019/01/RDD-FAQ-2019.pdf.

46 M. Salinsky, R. Kanter, and R. M. Dasheiff, "Effectiveness of Multiple EEGs in Supporting the Diagnosis of Epilepsy: An Operational Curve," *Epilepsia* 28, no. 4 (1987): 331–334, https://doi.org/10.1111/j.1528-1157.1987.tb03652.x.

47 Ipek Gurol-Urganci, Thyra de Jongh, Vlasta Vodopivec-Jamsek, Josip Car, and Rifat Atun, "Mobile Phone Messaging for Communicating Results of Medical Investigations," *Cochrane Database of Systematic Reviews* 6, (2012): CD007456, https://doi.org/10.1002/14651858.CD007456.pub2.

48 Maurice Flurie, Zachary Cline, Anne Marie Morse, Matthew Horsnell, Jennifer Gudeman, Lauryn Craine et al., "Beyond Brain Fog: A Social Listening Analysis of Impaired Cognitive Functioning in

Sleep Disorders," paper presented at Sleep 2024, Houston, TX, June 1–5, 2024, https://trend.community/wp-content/uploads/2024/05/SLEEP_2024_QR_Code.pdf.

49 "How We Work," TREND Community, accessed December 4, 2024, https://trend.community/how-we-work.

50 "Sleep Apnea Statistics and Facts You Should Know," National Council on Aging, October 9, 2024, https://www.ncoa.org/adviser/sleep/sleep-apnea-statistics/.

51 Ana Morelli, "Psychiatric Aspects of Chronic Physical Disease," *Medicine* 48, no. 12 (2020): 784–787, https://doi.org/10.1016/j.mpmed.2020.09.009, quoted in "Functional Disease," ScienceDirect, accessed December 4, 2024, https://www.sciencedirect.com/topics/medicine-and-dentistry/functional-disease.

52 Susannah Pick, Laura H. Goldstein, David L. Perez, and Timothy R. Nicholson, "Emotional Processing in Functional Neurological Disorder: A Review, Biopsychosocial Model and Research Agenda," *Journal of Neurology, Neurosurgery, and Psychiatry* 90, no. 6 (2019): 704–711, https://doi.org/10.1136/jnnp-2018-319201.

53 "National Statistics on Child Abuse," National Children's Alliance, accessed December 4, 2024, https://www.nationalchildrensalliance.org/media-room/old-national-statistics-on-child-abuse.

54 Ann Gold Buscho, "Divorce and Special Needs Children," *Psychology Today*, February 28, 2023, https://www.psychologytoday.com/intl/blog/a-better-divorce/202302/divorce-and-special-needs-children.

55 Aihui Chen, Yueming Pan, Longyu Li, and Yunshuang Yu, "Are You Willing to Forgive AI? Service Recovery from Medical AI Service Failure," *Industrial Management & Data Systems* 122, no. 11 (2022), https://doi.org/10.1108/IMDS-12-2021-0801.

56 Ekaterina Pesheva, "Does AI Help or Hurt Human Radiologists' Performance? It Depends on the Doctor," Harvard Medical School, March 2024, https://hms.harvard.edu/news/does-ai-help-or-hurt-human-radiologists-performance-depends-doctor.

57 Mohamed Khalifa and Mona Albadawy, "AI in Diagnostic Imaging: Revolutionising Accuracy and Efficiency," *Computer Methods and Programs in Biomedicine Update* 5 (2024): 100146, https://doi.org/10.1016/j.cmpbup.2024.100146.

58 Amardeep Rawat, "Top Healthcare Trends That Will Redefine the Industry in 2025," Appinventiv, December 27, 2024, https://appinventiv.com/blog/healthcare-app-trends.